Ingram
|17
30 —

P9-DHG-492

Marlborough Public Library
35 West Main Street
Marlborough, MA 01752

WHAT TO BELIEVE WHEN YOU'RE EXPECTING

WHAT TO BELIEVE WHEN YOU'RE EXPECTING

A New Look at Old Wives' Tales in Pregnancy

Jonathan Schaffir

ROWMAN & LITTLEFIELD
Lanham • Boulder • New York • London

Published by Rowman & Littlefield
A wholly owned subsidiary of The Rowman & Littlefield Publishing Group, Inc.
4501 Forbes Boulevard, Suite 200, Lanham, Maryland 20706
www.rowman.com

Unit A, Whitacre Mews, 26-34 Stannary Street, London SE11 4AB

Copyright © 2017 by Jonathan Schaffir

All rights reserved. No part of this book may be reproduced in any form or by any electronic or mechanical means, including information storage and retrieval systems, without written permission from the publisher, except by a reviewer who may quote passages in a review.

British Library Cataloguing in Publication Information Available

Library of Congress Cataloging-in-Publication Data

Names: Schaffir, Jonathan, 1965– author.
Title: What to believe when you're expecting : a new look at old wives' tales in pregnancy / Jonathan Schaffir.
Description: Lanham : Rowman & Littlefield, [2017] | Includes bibliographical references and index.
Identifiers: LCCN 2017007990 (print) | LCCN 2017012112 (ebook) | ISBN 9781538102084 (electronic) | ISBN 9781538102077 (cloth : alk. paper)
Subjects: LCSH: Pregnancy—Popular works.
Classification: LCC RG551 (ebook) | LCC RG551 .S33 2017 (print) | DDC 618.2—dc23

∞ ™ The paper used in this publication meets the minimum requirements of American National Standard for Information Sciences Permanence of Paper for Printed Library Materials, ANSI/NISO Z39.48-1992.

Printed in the United States of America

For Marcy, who believes in all the right things; and for Alison and Noah, who are the best proof of what makes a pregnancy turn out well.

CONTENTS

I

INTRODUCTION

As an obstetrician, I am used to all sorts of strange questions from my patients. When a woman has something that is nearly the size of a watermelon sitting squarely on top of her bladder and pelvic organs, no topics are off-limits. My day is peppered with all sorts of remarks about digestion, urination, back pain, swelling, and sex. In most cases, I have reasonable answers to these questions. After all, years of training and experience have provided me with insight into the problems that can crop up during pregnancy and the remedies that might be helpful. Even if I am not sure about the issue at hand, I know which textbook or journal to look in to find the answer.

Once in a while, I hear questions that are a bit more difficult to answer. These are the questions about issues that don't appear in medical textbooks. For example, a woman might ask me whether having sex or eating Chinese food will make her labor start sooner. Or whether drinking a beer will help her milk come in after delivery. A question I hear almost daily is whether you can tell if the baby will be a girl from how fast its heartbeat is. It would be easy to brush off these questions as silly or ill-informed. Why would spicy food start labor? There's no medical reason for that.

But it is not so easy to brush off these questions. For one thing, they keep popping up. They are not asked by just one person who might have gotten some strange notion in her head. They are voiced by dozens of women in my practice. When you hear the same suggestion over and over, you begin to think that maybe all those people suggesting it know something that you don't. Also, these questions are not proposed by poorly educated or eccentric women. They are expressed by women from all walks of life and all different cultures. When I ask them where they heard these notions, they often point to a trusted friend or an overbearing mother-in-law. No one ever tells me that they read about these issues in a patient handout or informational booklet.

Sometimes women speak of these recommendations earnestly. A woman frustrated by the discomfort of full-term pregnancy may be determined to find any reasonable way to get labor started a little sooner. Some of the information seems to be shared just for fun. Does anyone really think she can tell the baby's gender by swinging her wedding ring over her pregnant belly? Probably not, but it is an amusing diversion at a baby shower. Most of these suggestions are made in the same vein as the more serious questions about diet or vitamins or birthing classes. They originate from a sincere desire to find out what the baby will be like, how to care for it, and how to make the pregnancy easier.

Yet the types of recommendations and the individual pieces of advice are remarkably consistent. The idea that this information is being widely circulated without the aid of any official written directive is what earns them the term "obstetrical folklore." Like other pieces of folklore, they are communicated orally throughout a community, often over the course of generations. Since it is mostly women who talk about them, they are sometimes referred to as "old wives' tales," even though the sources are not necessarily old, and not necessarily married.

Now that everyone with a tablet or a smartphone can surf the Internet from anywhere in the world, such advice is more available and widespread than ever. Now a woman can find pages and pages of information about the most obscure pregnancy issues at the touch of a button. Providing this information has become easier, too. "Old wives" can post their opinions, experiences, and little-known facts on their personal webpages and blogs. Many websites have sprung up that offer advice on pregnancy, ranging from the sensible to the quite absurd. A simple Internet search will yield dozens of sites where women can purportedly determine the sex of their baby by entering the month of conception, or find a list of herbal remedies that will cure breast engorgement. There are also plenty of medically sound and well-researched sites that offer excellent advice to pregnant women about conception, pregnancy, and postpartum care. Yet even some reliable sources will share advice from "old wives," perhaps to entertain or to grab attention.

Although having access to this advice may be a product of the computer age, women may not realize that this wisdom is actually a relic of the Stone Age. Recommendations about getting pregnant and taking care of pregnancy have been around throughout recorded history, and probably as far back to when women could first use language to communicate about their birth experiences. What is surprising is how many of these tales exist on the Internet in almost the same form as they did in the writings of Hippocrates or in biblical times. There are few other types of advice that are passed on in all seriousness by seemingly authoritative web authors. For example, it would take a good deal of database searching to find a pediatric website where a parent recommends an ancient Greek remedy for an ear infection. But numerous hits will share a recipe for conceiving a male fetus that was formulated before the Christian era.

Most of these remedies are easily shrugged off as unscientific and unreasonable. A reasonably educated woman will probably not be convinced that attending a funeral might harm her baby. So why are all of these recommendations still being repeated in this age of evidence-based medical care? Is it purely for entertainment? What factors make pregnancy in particular such a (pardon the expression) fertile field for this advice to take hold? This book will sort through the many examples of such old wives' tales, from the ones that explain how to get pregnant quickly to the ones that help women recover from childbirth. It will try to explain why some remain popular and why they still get mentioned in doctors' offices routinely.

The term "folklore" implies that the information comes from a general sharing in the community, from common folk who are not necessarily experts. Unlike other types of advice and how-to writings, folklore can be passed along by anyone. Folklore is often associated with stories and information that is shared for entertainment and not necessarily for the purpose of improving one's health or well-being. But the subject of pregnancy is unique in the breadth and depth of folk advice that exists. Several factors conspire to make pregnancy unique in this regard.

Information about pregnancy is so commonly shared because pregnancy is so common. Although not every woman in the world will get pregnant, everyone has a mother, and most women will encounter someone who is pregnant at some point. And although many feel expert after going through this experience just once, many women can share opinions based on going through pregnancy multiple times. There are other bodily functions, of course, that are more universal, but not very many women are likely to share their advice and opinions about bowel movements, and discussing the ups and downs of menstruation is not considered appropriate for wide company.

Many people would lump advice about pregnancy together with recommendations about medical issues or treatments of disease. To find out how to diagnose a sore throat, or what to do for a twisted ankle, people turn to experts with letters after their names that demonstrate they have had medical training and would be expected to have special information about the treatment of illness. Even in ancient times, treatment of the ill was provided by members of the community who received special education and were regarded as healers. But unlike other medical issues, information about pregnancy has not traditionally been restricted to those with professional training. Historically, pregnant women have been taken care of by peers or elders with no special education. An older woman in the village does not need to understand the science of how a baby is conceived or what initiates the delivery process to have an opinion about how to get pregnant or start labor.

Pregnancy may also be viewed as a social rite or life event. People commonly share their opinions about various issues in life, from how to raise a child to how to deal with death. Pregnancy, however, is most often viewed as a joyous part of life, experienced when a woman is in her prime, and (usually) with a happy outcome. Women enjoy reliving their pregnancies and sharing their stories, and it is a topic that invites more discussion than coming of age rituals or old age. Unlike social events, though, the details of pregnancy are often beyond anyone's control. Both the timing and outcome are less certain than with social rituals such as marriage or retirement. Because the outcome of pregnancy is so uncertain, women may look for ways to control it and try to impose a happy ending. Advice about how to get pregnant quickly and guarantee a healthy baby would be very appealing.

Because the way that pregnancy turns out does not always follow a predictable pattern, most of the advice that has been passed down has very little impact on the actual outcome. Boys become boys and girls become girls regardless of what a woman eats or sleeps on. Labor starts at the appropriate time despite any number of activities to try to make it start sooner. Fortunately, the outcomes are generally good, so if the advice works, the recipient is happy; but even if it doesn't, she is still happy. Ironically, pregnancy advice may be the most commonplace because it so rarely has an effect.

Part of the appeal and longevity of such advice is due to the nature of pregnancy. But another aspect of the appeal is the recommendations themselves. The old wives' tales are often just that: stories. Like many stories, they can entertain, or make a point, or teach a lesson.

Many of the recommendations that were made in different time periods and in different cultures keep popping up because they are fun and entertaining. For example, the idea that a woman could affect what her unborn child looks like just by thinking about it seems like the stuff of fantasy. But for centuries, birth defects and markings were blamed on women's cravings, frights, or excitements. A story about a black woman having a white child because she saw a white statue when he was conceived dates back to the ancient Greeks, but it was also mentioned in the Middle Ages. Similar stories about children who were born with birthmarks that looked just like the strawberries that their mothers desired while pregnant occur in many different cultures. It may be preposterous to say that a child has a "harelip" because his mother was frightened by a rabbit during pregnancy. But the story keeps getting told because it is worth it to see the look of surprise and interest on the face of the woman who listens.

Sometimes these stories are told to justify or excuse behavior that might otherwise be frowned upon. A woman who constantly asks her husband to go and fetch her some sweet treat or weird combination of foods might start to get a reputation as something of a nag. But if the husband is convinced that refusing her wishes might end up damaging the baby, he will probably consider all those trips to the market worth it. Even adultery has been excused with such tales. A child that is born looking nothing like the supposed father might stir up all kinds of suspicions and accusations. The mother, however, might soothe her angry partner by explaining that she really was not doing anything wrong by just *looking* at the face of the milkman every day while she was pregnant. This idea of "maternal impression," that is, that babies are affected by their mother's thoughts, might get used again and again because of such advantages and not because the mother would really expect the link to hold up to scientific investigation.

Old wives' tales about maternal impression might also provide explanations for sad events that people do not understand and that their doctors could not explain. The first thought a woman has who miscarries or delivers a child with a birth defect is often "Why?" or more specifically, "Why me?" Her caregiver may not have any explanation other than that these things happen at random for no reason. The affected couple, however, might take some comfort in the idea that it was caused by a specific behavior or mental process. They might think that if the wife avoids attending a funeral the next time she is pregnant, then this won't happen again.

Wanting to impose a sense of purpose on events that cannot be easily explained or controlled is a strong factor in keeping pregnancy folklore going from one generation to the next. Although many couples would like to choose the exact month that they get pregnant, the process of conception occurs at random and often takes many months of trying. Naturally, waiting that long can lead to frustration, and a couple may start to look for ways that will bring the process under their control. Likewise, most women at the end of pregnancy are excited about the prospect of finally giving birth, but as the big day draws near, they might become anxious and start to worry. When will labor start? Is the pain as bad as everyone says? Will there be complications? Believing that there are ways to control the onset of labor or minimize pain gives women a sense of empowerment that goes a long way in reducing their anxiety. The advice that a woman gets may work or it may fail, but either way it helps her to feel less frightened and more in charge of an event that is impossible to control.

Mostly, however, recommendations keep getting passed on because the women who share them think they will work. If women were told to follow a particular pregnancy diet, and none of the women who did got pregnant, it is safe to say the recommendation would not last very long. Of course, some women will get pregnant regardless of what they are eating. About half of the women who take that special concoction to have a boy will conceive a boy no matter what advice they follow. The fact that favorable outcomes occur routinely makes it seem like such recommendations are having the intended effect. Women who make the link between following pregnancy advice and having the desired outcome don't have the perspective to know whether they got what they wanted due to cause and effect, or just by happenstance.

If all these outcomes do just happen at random, it still seems remarkable that certain advice regarding pregnancy has remained so consistent from one generation to the next, or across different cultures. For example, if breast milk comes in naturally no matter what kind of diet a woman follows, then you might expect all kinds of remedies to be offered for decreased breast milk. But the idea of drinking beer to increase milk production has appeared in writings from ancient Egypt to Victorian England to the modern Internet. Why would one particular piece of advice be so consistent? Perhaps in some cases the advice persists because it really does work. Perhaps the ancient naturalists noticed a pattern in which women were likely to conceive boys, or who would miscarry, or when labor would start. Maybe these early observers paid such close attention to the outcomes of their "experiments" that they uncovered new information about the nature of pregnancy. In other words, maybe the old wives were right.

Proving whether these ideas are correct or incorrect has inspired a large amount of scientific research. Whether they find it ridiculous and want to prove it wrong, or whether they hope there might be some useful truth among the old wives' tales, scientists have devoted significant time and effort to research on this kind of folklore. Proving that a piece of advice might really have the desired effect on pregnancy can be very difficult. The best way for a scientific study to determine if there is a true cause-and-effect relationship between a behavior and a result is with a therapeutic trial. In this type of research, one group is given a particular therapy or intervention (like a medicine or an activity), while an identical group is given a placebo or no therapy. The researchers would then count the number of subjects who had the outcome they were looking for. Presumably if more people who used the intervention had the desired outcome than the people who did not, then it would be safe to say that taking that medicine or engaging in that activity helped to bring about the desired effect. Doing this kind of research on pregnancy folklore, however, is not so easy. Some of the interventions that are mentioned, like having sex or giving in to cravings, are difficult to give up for the sake of an experiment. Other interventions like ingesting herbs or restricting diets might be potential sources of harm, and it would be unethical to ask pregnant women to participate. Sometimes it is just not feasible to design a trial that would prove a cause and effect.

Take for example one particular old wives' tale about getting labor to start. One piece of advice given by ancient Greeks to bring on contractions was to lift the pregnant woman and drop her onto a couch. The concept of assisting labor by repetitive pounding or bouncing was still written about through the Middle Ages and during the Renaissance. Though bouncing a laboring woman up and down sounds a little sadistic, it is not very different from the recommendation that can still be heard today: bringing on labor by having a woman drive over a bumpy road. Might this practice have persisted because it is effective? This would not be an easy test to undertake because it would be very difficult to control the amount of strain that a woman would have to endure, and no researcher is likely to take this on as a personal project. More importantly, no group of pregnant women would agree to have the theory tested because it would certainly be uncomfortable and may cause harm.

Other examples of folklore may not be the subject of research projects because they lack biological plausibility. In other words, if there is no good reason to think that a particular piece of advice would have a biological effect on pregnancy, then it probably will not be tested. Since ancient times, people have worn and worshipped fertility symbols, including charms, amulets, and images. Some women today still admit to carrying such a charm during their efforts at conceiving. But there will probably never be a research study that prospectively records the pregnancy outcomes of women carrying charms and those who don't because no one in the scientific community is likely to believe this would have a true cause and effect.

Nevertheless, there are enough recommendations out there that sound just rational enough to be true, or where a positive effect was seen frequently enough to pique someone's curiosity. Consequently, a substantial body of scientific literature has been written to either support or refute the suspicions that these recommendations are worth following. Some of this research consists of reliable, well-reasoned studies that carefully measure the effects of folk interventions. Others are less rigorous or more biased, and their conclusions deserve to be taken with a grain of salt.

In this book, I have brought together and analyzed the evidence for or against the bulk of obstetrical folklore. Not every type of pregnancy folklore has been put under the researcher's microscope, and not all of the research that has been done is useful for the average woman interested in everyday advice. Most of what I've included are the persistent themes: the types of advice that keep popping up in more than one culture and why they are repeated. Often these recommendations keep recurring not because they really work, but because they sound plausible or entertaining.

The entire range of pregnancy advice is included, from directions on how best to get pregnant through recommendations on getting through the postpartum period. The folklore mentioned here is generally restricted to Western society, in large part because what is written about this subject in English deals mostly with European and American cultures. Folklore by definition depends on the society from which it arises and the folks who talk about it. Beliefs about pregnancy may be very different in various parts of the world. In an American suburban medical office, many women are educated and will not take old wives' tales seriously. In developing countries where women lack access to education, discussion of spirits and environmental influences may take on much greater importance. Anthropologists who travel around the world to observe the indigenous peoples of the Amazon River basin or the tribes of Papua New Guinea have brought back very interesting stories about their pregnancy practices and beliefs. These are generally not the sorts of discussions that will typically be overheard in the waiting room of the average American obstetrician. Occasionally, there is some overlap between what has been described in nonindustrialized cultures and what is read on the Internet, and trying to explain how such advice found its way from one to the other proves interesting.

The primary focus of this book, though, is on those recommendations that are commonly discussed in modern Western culture. These are the practices that have most extensively been researched and investigated by physicians and sociologists. Likewise, they are the ones most likely to be shared between women who are looking online for advice on pregnancy. Searching online for interesting tidbits about pregnancy advice may be a fun and entertaining way to pass some time during those long hours of waiting for a baby to arrive. But if a woman is wondering which of those tidbits might really help her and what might be a waste of her time, this book will help to guide her exploration.

2

GETTING PREGNANT

For many (if not most) women, getting pregnant happens all too easily. Whether it is the eager newlywed or the less-than-careful teenager, a woman has a few episodes of unprotected intercourse and that stick she bought at the drugstore turns blue. For some women, however, getting pregnant can be a source of tremendous anxiety and stress. Many couples struggle for years with unsuccessfully trying to get pregnant. The urge to have children is such a powerful human desire that when this demand can't be met, it can cause frustration and even depression. Sometimes the frustration is not from years of trying to get pregnant, but just from a perceived delay because nature's timetable doesn't always mesh with a woman's plans. Regardless, that sense of urgency to conceive motivates many women to look for help when nature isn't cooperating. Women looking for help with getting "in a family way" will find no shortage of suggestions for how to do it from their friends and families.

The idea of looking for outside influences to help improve the chance of conceiving is as old as humankind itself. Some of the earliest pieces of sculpture found are thought to be fertility charms dating back twenty thousand years before our era. The most famous of these, the "Venus of Willendorf," is thought to be one of the earliest known representations of the human form. Many similar figurines have been found across Eurasia, all dating from the Stone Age. The vast majority of these depict women, and usually nude. [1]

What would lead archaeologists to think these are fertility idols? The majority of them depict women with oversize breasts, thighs, and buttocks. Coming from a time when food was generally scarce it is unlikely that the majority of women were obese; these representations are thought to be a more idealized form of womanhood, one that would be associated with greater fertility. In later cultures, too, statues of goddesses that were associated with fertility had exaggerated or prominent breasts. A statue of the Greek goddess Artemis, a fertility deity, was even depicted as having multiple rows of breasts![2]

Sexual characteristics are similarly exaggerated for idols associated with male fertility.[3] Ancient Greeks who were having difficulty conceiving a child sought help and prayed to gods that were thought to be particularly manly and virile. These gods, such as Pan and Priapus, were often depicted with ridiculously large penises, signifying their potency and ability to inspire fertility and sexual prowess. African fertility idols are also seen that feature supersized penises. Such oversize depictions of the male member are seen not just on idols, but on charms and amulets that are thought to improve chances of getting a woman pregnant.

So were these depictions just wishful thinking, or is there really some connection between large sexual organs and fertility? Several studies have examined penile size in populations of men and compared it with other personal characteristics.[4] Although none of them look specifically at number of pregnancies or sperm count, there have been comparisons to testicular volume, which relates to sperm production. Despite what the ancient Greeks might have men believe, there is no relationship between penis size and the volume of the testicle. So it would appear that having a larger member does not necessarily make a man more likely to get a woman pregnant.

What about the female side? Why would the ancient sculptors who were trying to inspire women to get pregnant carve idols with large breasts and buttocks? It is possible that it was just an overemphasized attention to sexual organs, the way that they also drew attention to the penis. But studies that measure the hormones that go along with ovulation in large groups of women have shown that women are more likely to ovulate regularly (and therefore get pregnant) if they have low waist-to-hip ratios. That is, bigger hips and smaller waists suggest a greater pregnancy potential than small hips and a wide waist. One study that also looked at breast size found the greatest potential for fertility among those women who had wider hips and also larger breasts.[5] So those ancient artists and sculptors may have been on to something.

Nowadays, there are still women who carry charms or amulets to help them conceive. Most of the time, this practice is associated with non-Western cultures; there are not many women in the average reproductive specialist's office wearing a figurine of an obese woman. Any woman who goes Internet shopping for such a pendant, however, will likely find several examples of full-figured figurines that are sold to improve chances of getting pregnant. There is never likely to be a study involving women who wear such amulets, but they may be interested to know that their purchases may have been inspired by a kernel of truth.

Other examples of folklore advice that women share about trying to get pregnant are based on elements in nature that are associated with fertility. Women frustrated with infertility have looked at the world around them and noted that certain animals or plants seem to reproduce very easily, and these must hold secrets to easy conception. Since many superstitions are based on the idea that ingesting or being near a thing with a desired quality will give the bearer the same desired quality, many pieces of advice involve fertility tokens. Anything perceived to produce many offspring or resemble offspring may be involved in fertility superstitions.

Eggs have been associated with fertility in many cultures, due to the obvious connection between producing an egg and producing young. Some cultures advocate ingesting eggs, while others encourage their decoration or adornment as symbols of fertility. Fish are also viewed as fertile beings, probably because of the large numbers of eggs that they spawn, and eating fish is another common recommendation that women are given to help conceive.[6]

Perhaps no animal is more linked to fertility than the rabbit. It is no accident that the expression "breeding like rabbits" has come into use since these animals do indeed have a large number of offspring. Not surprisingly, rabbits are often involved in fertility lore. An Anglo-Saxon belief involves tying a rabbit bone around a woman's abdomen to help her conceive. This seems considerably more palatable than an ancient Greek recipe that called for women to conceive by drinking a broth made from the pulverized womb of a hare.[7] Interestingly, the practice of eating rabbit uterus has also been cited in modern-day Turkey. A survey of women attending a family planning center in the city of Van in 2009 included a few who sampled this tidbit just before intercourse in order to get pregnant.[8] Unfortunately, this study did not say whether the women who did so got pregnant more easily. While not quite as fertile as rabbits, dogs are also noted to have large litters of pups. Ancient Greeks thus also advocated for eating meat from man's best friend to help women conceive.[9]

The prospect of eating such unappealing meat dishes may have led other women to try vegetarian approaches to a fertility diet; the food-stuffs may be considered more palatable but the principle is the same. Plants that grow with multiple small seeds are often viewed as being more fertile and would therefore give whoever eats them greater powers of fertility. Rice, which grows on stalks that are loaded with lots of individual seeds, has long been seen as a fertility aid. The practice of throwing rice at newlyweds at weddings began as a practice to encourage a fruitful union. Pomegranates and figs have also been included in fertility-enhancing recipes, presumably because of their seed-filled qualities.

Women of today are less likely to be taken in by the simple idea that "like begets like," meaning that a person can attain the same quality of another substance just by eating it or being near it. Nevertheless, there is quite an industry that has arisen in recommending foods that will promote fertility. Various books and websites promote variations on a "fertility diet" that will improve the odds of conception. Beans, pumpkin seeds, pineapple, and even baby carrots (for babies, of course) have been recommended as foods that will enhance attempts at pregnancy. Some websites offer to sell specific recipes and diets that they promise will succeed in yielding that longed-for baby. Most of these sites are run by hucksters who prey on gullible and desperate women who have been unsuccessful trying more mainstream methods.

For most women, there is no reason to think that what she eats will change the way her body readies itself for reproduction to any great extent. The period of time during which a woman can conceive occurs for just a few days each month around the time that she ovulates (that is, when the ovary releases an egg). When conception does not occur, a menstrual period follows about two weeks later. For women who report having regular periods that occur each month, it is usually a safe bet that they are ovulating regularly and should be able to get pregnant.

There is no reason to think that eating a certain food or diet will change that pattern.

In some women, periods are irregular, and this may be a sign that ovulation is not occurring on a monthly basis. These women may have more difficulty getting pregnant, and changes that would affect menstrual regularity could affect chances for conception. Such irregularity is most likely to occur at extremes of weight, with both very underweight women and obese women having problems with less frequent ovulation. It is easier to imagine how a change of diet in these populations could improve fertility.

One group of scientists did investigate the diets of women who had difficulty conceiving because of irregular ovulation.[10] They followed more than seventeen thousand women over the course of eight years as they tried to become pregnant. They compared the diets of women who became pregnant and those who did not, and particularly paid attention to the women whose infertility was linked to not ovulating regularly. They found that the women who had trouble getting pregnant were more likely to follow diets that were high in trans fats, carbohydrates with a high glycemic index (that is, rapidly absorbed simple sugars), and animal proteins. They also noted that women who did not routinely take a multivitamin had more difficulty in getting pregnant.[11]

The conclusion of these researchers is that following a healthy diet (by limiting sweets and fried foods, consuming a moderate amount of animal meat, and getting sufficient vitamins) will maximize the chance of getting pregnant. They didn't actually prove that following this "pregnancy diet" will cause an infertile woman to get pregnant more easily. It may be that women who eat lots of candy and hamburgers also have other bad habits that contribute to infertility, or maybe an unhealthy diet also has a bad effect on their sex life. In any case, these findings are not surprising, given that health in general contributes to fertility and a healthy pregnancy. The evidence falls short of proving that a particular diet can lead to pregnancy, but it certainly sounds like a good idea for women trying to get pregnant to maintain a healthy weight and a healthy body.

There is no particular food item that is likely to make a woman ovulate more regularly, but some herbal remedies have been recommended for that purpose. The most common remedy mentioned by women trying herbal preparations to get pregnant is the chasteberry, or *vitex agnus*. The chasteberry gets its name because it is a fruit that is rumored to help its consumer remain chaste.[12] According to old lore, chasteberry was recommended for modest women who might be led astray by their sexual longings and for monks who needed help getting rid of sexual urges to remain celibate. No studies have ever proven that the chasteberry is actually useful for suppressing sexual desire, though.[13] It is unclear when the association with fertility emerged, but this seems to be a more modern recommendation.

There is little evidence that eating a lot of chasteberry will overcome infertility. However, one study of a nutritional supplement containing a chasteberry extract showed some promising results.[14] The supplement combined this extract with vitamins and antioxidants like green tea and l-arginine, so it is uncertain exactly what component had the greatest effect. The product was given to fifty-three women who had been trying unsuccessfully to get pregnant for at least six months, and another forty women were given a placebo. After three months, 26 percent of the group taking the chasteberry extract were pregnant, compared with only 10 percent of the placebo group. This may not be characterized as an overwhelming success, but it suggests that this particular extract may be helpful for women looking for a little boost in their fertility.

The folklore surrounding diets and particular foods are thought to work by helping women ovulate more regularly. Because irregular ovulation is just one of many reasons why it might be difficult to get pregnant, it makes sense that remedies aimed toward improving ovulation are not going to work all the time. Particularly when it comes to the everyday people who pass on folklore advice, they are not thinking about ovulation. They are thinking primarily about what it takes to have a baby: the sex act itself. It is no surprise, then, that much of the advice about getting pregnant quickly and easily centers on the when and how of having sex.

Advice about the sexual act existed even before people understood just how conception occurred. It was not until the seventeenth century that the early microscopists looked at semen under a microscope and identified spermatozoa, and after seeing these tiny cells swimming around decided that they were the necessary ingredient to get a woman with child. However, semen was always known to be necessary for conception, and ancient physicians figured that it somehow contained the necessary "seed" that needed to be planted in the woman's fertile "field." Paulus of Aegina in the seventh century advised couples to have coitus after dinner and in bed, because the woman falling asleep would be more likely to keep the male seed inside of her.[15] Ambrose Pare, a sixteenth-century physician, gave similar advice: he recommended that women should hold still after intercourse, remain silent, and keep their legs elevated to hold the semen in place. He also advised that men should delay removing the penis from the vagina so that no air would enter and "modify the seed." He also suggested that conception would be more likely to occur if both parties were sexually satisfied, and went so far as to recommend that the husband should stimulate the wife's genitals to make sure that she is adequately pleasured since this would aid with conception.

The idea of remaining in a certain position in order to give semen the longest possible time to remain in contact with the vagina remains common today. Many couples claim to have been told that the "missionary position" is best for getting pregnant, since having the woman beneath the man will prevent the semen from running out. Another frequent recommendation is for the woman to lie still for a while after sex with a towel or a pillow underneath her hips in order to prevent spillage. Whether this practice really gives any advantage to the couple trying to conceive is questionable. Plenty of babies have been born into this world following couplings of their parents in all sorts of positions that defy the effects of gravity. There have not been any studies that look at fertility rates for couples in various sexual positions, and there are not likely to be, since few couples would agree to take part in a study where intercourse had to take place in the same position month after month.

As for whether enhancing female sexual pleasure could make it easier to conceive, those ancient doctors may have been onto something. There are indeed changes in the vaginal anatomy during lovemaking that bring semen into closer and longer contact with the woman's cervix.[16] Masters and Johnson were the first to study and describe how the human vagina changes during coitus. They outfitted women with various monitors and pressure gauges while having sex or pleasuring themselves in order to see just what transpired during the various phases of genital stimulation. They noted that during arousal, which they term the "excitement phase," the upper part of the vagina relaxes and expands while the muscles at the outer part of the vagina begin to contract and make the vaginal opening narrower. This results in a reservoir near the cervix where semen can collect, and makes it harder for the semen to spill out. Others have noted that the fluid that lubricates the vagina when a woman becomes aroused can serve as a buffer, letting the more alkaline semen survive in the normally acidic environment of the vagina. This lubricant also increases the amount of oxygen available to sperm cells, which allows more sperm to survive.[17] Orgasm involves vaginal and uterine contractions that may also play a role in helping to get sperm into the cervix and through the uterus. It has not been proven that a woman is more likely to conceive in a sex act where she climaxes compared with one where she does not. Still, as recommendations about getting pregnant go, this one may be the most appealing.

Another very common piece of advice shared with couples trying to conceive is to make sure that the concentration and potency of the man's ejaculate is as strong as it can be. Men often hear advice that having sex too often will result in sperm counts that are too low to result in pregnancy, by using up the limited supply of their little swimmers too quickly. The caution not to have sex too often may date back to ancient times, and in the sixteenth century Pare was also telling men to wait a little while between acts of sex so that the semen would be thick and "full of lively spirits."[18] Whereas Pare might have thought of semen as actually containing little ghosts, we now think of those spirits as being sperm cells. Sperm are produced constantly in the male testicle, so there is always a new supply being made. Still many men fear that their supply is in danger of being used up if they ejaculate too often. Various sources claim that a couple will improve their chance of conception by having sex every other day rather than daily. In fact, the male testicle is a fairly efficient sperm factory, and ejaculation daily may decrease the volume but not the concentration of sperm in most men.[19] Since each time that a couple has sex increases the chance that they will get pregnant, it is hard to say just where the balance lies between too much and too little sex. It is probably safe to say that a couple does not have to take breaks from having sex just to increase the man's potency, but since assigned sex on particular days may be stressful and unromantic, they may choose to take a break here and there for other reasons.

Something else that may have an adverse effect on sperm count is a rise in temperature. It has long been known that the testicle does not produce sperm as well when it is overheated. Tests that measure sperm production in men with fever show a reduced count, as do research studies that have subjected their participants to artificial heating of the scrotum.[20] This effect has led men to believe that they will have the best chance of getting a woman pregnant if they wear clothing that will keep their testicles cool. In particular, wearing boxers instead of briefs is thought to allow the testes to get plenty of air by letting them hang away from the body. Although this advice is a feature only of modern times, the boxers versus briefs debate has become so frequently voiced that it has entered the realm of fertility folklore. In fact, scientists have examined this piece of advice by comparing sperm counts in men wearing briefs with those who wear boxers.[21] The study showed that boxers did indeed result in a higher concentration of sperm. Whether it is enough to increase chances of conception, however, is debatable.

All the talk about what to eat, what to wear, and how to have sex is enough to make any couple get a bit tense. In contrast to all this regimentation, another common piece of advice that couples often hear for achieving pregnancy is to relax. Couples struggling with infertility often hear stories about friends or relatives who tried and tried to get pregnant, using all kinds of medical and nonmedical assistance, only to fail despite their efforts. It is only after giving up and quitting the stress of putting their love life under the microscope that they suddenly conceive, with no help at all! Although this sort of happy ending no doubt occurs from time to time, it is probably not as common as people would like to believe.

Nevertheless, infertility is undoubtedly a stressful and frustrating situation. Trying unsuccessfully to conceive is associated with increased rates of depression and anxiety, and can have detrimental effects on relationships leading to anger between partners and ultimately breakup or divorce. Stress is also recognized as having direct effects on various bodily functions, leading to increased susceptibility to illness, digestive problems, and abnormal menstrual cycles. Since stress can have such an impact on both the mind and the body, it would make sense that it may also make it more difficult for a woman to get pregnant. In fact, studies do demonstrate an effect of mental stress on fertility.[22] Women undergoing infertility procedures such as intrauterine insemination (where semen is injected directly into the uterus) and in vitro fertilization (where the egg is fertilized outside of the body and then transferred back into the uterus) were administered questionnaires to see how they were feeling at the time they had these procedures. These fertility procedures were less likely to be successful in those women with the highest depression and anxiety scores.

It would follow that practices that reduce stress levels may therefore improve chances of conception. There are many techniques that are known to reduce stress, and some of those that have been suggested to improve the chances of conceiving include yoga, meditation, massage, hypnosis, and mindfulness.[23] Some of these complementary and alternative treatments have been studied in women who were having difficulty getting pregnant. Although such practices have been shown to decrease stress and contribute to a general sense of well-being, no studies have demonstrated higher rates of conception or more successful in vitro fertilization procedures. Even so, there may be other downstream benefits of such treatments. Some advocates have suggested that when physicians advocate for stress reduction activities on behalf of their patients, it may improve patients' trust in their doctors and lead to improved communication.

Acupuncture is a complementary therapeutic practice that has been adopted from the East but recommended more and more commonly in Western cultures to enhance fertility. It is hard for doctors trained in Western medicine to understand just how sticking needles into a woman would have a positive effect on her fertility. Practitioners of acupuncture claim that it may have a relaxing effect, so the mechanism may be by reducing stress. Although the other stress reduction techniques mentioned above have not been closely examined, several studies have looked at the use of acupuncture in women undergoing fertility treatment. One group of authors collected the results of several of these studies to demonstrate the effect of acupuncture in the entire number of women who were studied.[24] With this large pool, they demonstrated that women who were undergoing in vitro fertilization were more likely to have a successful procedure if they also used acupuncture as an adjunct to their medical treatment. This effect has not been shown as convincingly in women who were trying to conceive naturally without the medical treatment. So the advice to relax is not necessarily proven to help the average woman get pregnant. Nevertheless, for those women stressed by complicated fertility treatments like in vitro fertilization, any complementary treatment that can be calming and contribute to mental well-being could benefit efforts at conception.

When all else fails and frustration mounts, it is common for women to call on the help of a higher power. The idea of fertility being controlled by a deity or supernatural being is probably as old as humankind itself. In ancient times, people worshipped many gods, with each one assigned a particular province or specialty that would be an area of importance to their worshippers. Since food was crucial to survival, every culture had a god representing the hunt or the fields, and prayers to those gods would ensure food on the table. Since expanding the family was also crucial to the survival of the culture, each society also assigned a deity to be in charge of fertility. Examples of prayers to fertility deities can be found in nearly every culture. In fact, one of the earliest examples of human writing, a cuneiform tablet from Sumer dating back to about 3000 BCE, features an invocation to a god of childbirth.[25] Usually, the deity assigned to fertility was a goddess, and she was the one to whom women would pray and make offerings in the hope that it would help them to have a child. In ancient Mesopotamia, it was Ishtar, whom the Phoenicians referred to as Astarte. The ancient Sumerians prayed to the fertility goddess Inanna, and the Etruscans sought help from Mater Matuta. The Egyptians had Isis, and the Greeks prayed to Aphrodite, though Hera and Artemis also received their share of prayers from barren women seeking help.

Even as times changed and more people began to adopt the idea of a Judeo-Christian God, prayers to assist with childbearing were just as common even though only a single god was involved. The Bible has several stories of women having difficulty conceiving but whose prayers were rewarded in due time. Sarah conceived Isaac in her nineties after being visited by angels who promised that she would conceive, and Hannah had similar success with the birth of Samuel.

Even today, prayer remains a common practice for women who have difficulty conceiving. Women attending a Midwestern fertility clinic were surveyed about the nonmedical methods they used in addition to standard treatments in order to help them get pregnant.[26] Forty-eight percent listed prayer as an alternative or complementary therapy, which was the most common one identified. A survey of Chinese men diagnosed with infertility revealed that many attend temples to pray that they will be able to have children, since they become frustrated with the lack of results they get from Western medicine.[27] Men and women diagnosed with infertility may feel that they are dealing with a crisis, and prayer and spirituality offer them a source of comfort and support. Prayer is also an expression of hope, and people worship so that their prayers for children may be granted.

It is easy to recognize why people would pray when they want to have a baby, but it would be very hard to prove that prayer could actually improve the chance of conceiving. In order to show that any treatment has an effect, scientists ideally look to a group of people with identical circumstances where some have the treatment and some do not, and then see if there is a difference in their outcome. Prayer is a very difficult intervention to control, since a researcher would be hard-pressed to say that two infertile couples are the same in every way but that one prayed more.

Nevertheless, at least one study has been done to try to prove that prayer can affect a woman's chances of getting pregnant.[28] In the experiment, a church group in the United States was given pictures of the faces of a random selection of Korean women undergoing in vitro fertilization. The church group was given the assignment of intercessory prayer, or praying on behalf of the pictured women that they would conceive. The researchers then compared the success rate in the group of women whose pictures were shared and the group of women for whom no praying had occurred. As originally published, the authors state that the group of women whose pictures were prayed over conceived twice as frequently as women undergoing in vitro fertilization whose pictures were not sent.

The study generated considerable controversy. It was widely publicized at first, since it seemed to demonstrate the power of prayer. However, it received more publicity for its questionable methods. First there were concerns over an invasion of privacy, since the women involved did not consent to having their pictures prayed over or having strangers know that they were going through infertility treatments. There were also questions about how the results were counted and whether the research was done honestly. One author withdrew his name from the study shortly after publication and another was convicted of fraud. The journal eventually withdrew the paper from circulation, since the publishers would not stand behind a study whose results were tainted by such questionable methodology and possible fraud.[29] So there has not yet been a study to unequivocally prove the power of prayer in enhancing fertility. It is unlikely that an unbiased study on the subject will be possible. Even if it is not proven, however, many infertile couples will continue to pray for children since there is no downside. And who knows? It may even help.

It is also, perhaps, the easiest to accomplish of the many and varied tips that people have offered to overcome infertility. Some of these tips, like the advice to eat certain organ meats, may be unappealing and rarely followed. Other advice, like directions about sex positions, is easier to follow and may even be pleasurable. Still, there are some common themes that ring true. Couples hoping to conceive are advised to eat healthy, relax, enjoy the process, have faith, and hope for a positive outcome. In any guise, these are recommendations that anyone can follow.

3

CHOOSING A BABY'S GENDER*

Of all the characteristics that their future child may have, the one that parents fixate on the most is the baby's gender. Despite the fifty–fifty odds that nature presents in selecting baby's sex, parents since antiquity have looked for ways to influence this outcome. Since most Western societies through history place more value on male children and pass all of their inheritances to sons, the search has usually been for ways to produce male offspring. Whether because of royalty looking to produce male heirs or poor workers trying to avoid paying large dowries for daughters, the majority of recommendations for choosing fetal sex involve having a boy baby. Many couples, however, are motivated by a desire to produce a child of the sex opposite of the children they already have. The mother raising three boys, for example, is often desperate for a trick to ensure the next child will be a girl. Regardless of motivation, the wish to have a child of a particular gender has resulted in a host of recipes and techniques for sex selection through the ages.

*According to some, "sex" is biologically determined by the baby's genitalia, but "gender" is a psychological construct, meaning that a biologically male individual may identify as female or something in between. For the purpose of this book, however, I am using the two terms interchangeably, since this is how the majority of people use the terms in everyday parlance. And because expectant parents aren't generally trying to choose or predict the psychological mindset of their babies, just what the genitalia will look like!

Some of the oldest recommendations for sex selection revolve around the idea that one side of the body favors males while the other favors females. In antiquity, the right side of the body was assigned characteristics that were associated with masculinity. Because most people are right-handed, the right was perceived as stronger and more skilled, while the left hand was more often weak and awkward. The word "dextrous" comes from the Latin *dexter*, meaning right, and still has a positive and desirable connotation. The Latin word for left, on the other hand, is *sinister*, a word that we have come to think of as negative and undesirable. Since men in the male-dominated society were perceived to be stronger and dominant, it seemed natural to the ancients that they should come from the right side of the body.

Ancient Greek medicine also described health and illness as a balance of hot and cold humors. Men, having greater strength and power, were believed to have more natural heat. The ancients thus believed that a baby growing in a place that would offer more heat would naturally turn into a boy. As Hippocrates wrote, "Males, inclined to fire, grow from foods and regimen that are dry and warm."[1] Because the liver, which lies on the right side of the body, was viewed as a "hot" organ, it was thought that the right side of the uterus would furnish more of the heat necessary to nourish a male fetus. In the fifth century BCE, Parmenides suggested that a woman could ensure the birth of a son by lying on her right side immediately after intercourse to allow the seed to settle there.[2] Now, even twenty-five hundred years later, one can still find women on chat rooms on the Internet telling each other that they can increase the chance of having a boy by lying on the right side during or after having sex.

Even though the baby was known to grow in the woman and be affected by the qualities of her womb, the distinction between left and right side was applied to the male partner as well. Since men have two testicles and there are two possible genders, ancient naturalists figured that would mean that one testicle supplied a "male seed" that led to boys, and the other a "female seed" that produced girls. Again, the right side was viewed as the source for male seed. Galen, a Roman physician writing in the second century CE, described the anatomical reasoning behind this concept. He pointed out that on the right side of the body, the veins attached to the testicles and ovaries connect directly to the inferior vena cava, the big central vein that leads to the heart. On the left side, however, these same veins connect not with the vena cava, but with the renal veins, making a little detour toward the kidneys. He wrote that, as a result, "the left testis in the male and the left uterus in the female receive blood still uncleansed, full of residues, watery and serous, and so it happens that the . . . instruments on the right side, nourished with pure blood, become warmer than those on the left."[3] This greater natural heat would be more likely to produce male offspring. What Galen did not realize at the time was that the veins don't bring nourishment to the organs, but instead carry blood away from the organs. It would take another fifteen hundred years before William Harvey would show that blood circulates around the body in one direction, with the arteries supplying the organs with fresh blood and the veins bringing away waste. And as it happens, both the testicular and ovarian arteries come from the same central artery on both sides of the body.

In the seventeenth century, the French obstetrician Francois Mauriceau pointed this out, demonstrating that the blood that is carried to the sex organs is exactly the same on both sides. He used this anatomical fact to refute some of his colleagues who were so convinced that the right testicle produced male sperm that they recommended tying off, or even cutting off, the left testicle in order to conceive boys. Furthermore, he related the case of an Italian acquaintance who had only one testicle, but who fathered a child of each sex without "the assistance of any other in that business."[4]

Just as those physicians of yesteryear reasoned that one testicle must be responsible for each gender, there were some who reasoned that the ovaries could have a similar assignment. Within another hundred years when the egg cell was identified as coming from the ovary, some theorized that whichever side the ovum came from played a role in determining gender. Well into the nineteenth century, some physicians proposed that the one ovary would only produce girl eggs and the other ovary would yield boys. As abdominal surgery became a more common occurrence in the late nineteenth century, surgeons were able to demonstrate that women who had had an ovary removed were still able to conceive children of either gender. Even today, there are women who can feel which side they ovulate on, and think that they can tell their child's gender based on where they felt ovulation pain at the time of conception. In the scientific mainstream, though, the right–left theories of gender origin have been abandoned, and they remain only the stuff of old wives' tales.

Another line of thinking that keeps popping up over the years is the idea that male gender is a product of male virility. The "like breeds like" attitude has led many would-be parents to assume that more manly men are more likely to produce male children. An early eighteenth-century physician put it like this: "Weakly men get most girls, if they get any children at all."[5] This line of thinking is still heard today, by folks who observe that couples where the man is more dominant are more likely to have boys than girls. Some even go so far as to recommend that women who want to conceive a male child should be submissive in the bedroom and let their sexual partners be more dominant.

Perhaps this type of thinking is still voiced because there have been some interesting observations over the years that make it seem somewhat reasonable. Most of the support for this theory comes from population studies, where information about a society or community is explored by looking at large registries or databases. A social scientist trying to see if particular characteristics of that society influence the gender of offspring would look at the sex ratio of the population. The sex ratio is the proportion of male babies to female babies in a given time frame. If the chance of having a boy is always fifty–fifty, one would expect the sex ratio to be exactly one, meaning that for every one hundred males born, there are also one hundred females born. (Actually, a normal sex ratio is slightly greater than one, since most populations generate about fifty-one boys for every forty-nine girls. Some have argued this is because boys are not as likely to survive as girls, or that men die earlier, so the ratio of adult sexes is always about equal.) Still, a sex ratio that is significantly higher than one would invite questions about what happened to make boys more commonly born during that period.

In the early nineteenth century, a sociologist compiling statistics from the register of British peerage noticed that the sex ratio fell as the difference in age of spouses grew.[6] Specifically, for men and women of equal age, the chance of having a boy or girl was fairly equal. However, men considerably older than their wives were much more likely to have male children. For men younger than their wives, the opposite was true; girl babies were more common. This author suggested that these differences were caused by the older men being more dominant, and therefore having a male-like influence over their spouses.

Several nineteenth-century papers quote similar statistics.[7] Some used absolute rather than relative ages, but again concluded that the gender of offspring is influenced by which parent is more mature. One author demonstrated this to be true until the male partner approached age fifty, when the ratio became more equal again. He felt that this was likely because aging men start to lose their strength and stamina, and so they at some point are less capable of influencing the baby's gender in the male direction.

Studies looking at sex ratios related to war have demonstrated that the ratio of male to female babies has been greatest in the time periods just after World Wars I and II.[8] For people who believe that male dominance can influence a baby's gender, this observation is doubly relevant. First, these periods were associated with greater mean age differences in married couples, since women were more likely to wed older men when the younger male population was depleted by war. Secondly, the men who did fight and survived the war long enough to reproduce may have been stronger and better able to defend themselves during wartime conflict.

More recent studies also suggest higher male to female ratios in couples where the woman is a victim of domestic violence, or even in pregnancies that are a result of rape.[9] In these cases, the imbalance of power is more literal, with women being overpowered by men who may be not only physically dominant, but violent as well. It remains to be seen whether characteristics like virility, strength, or violent tendencies are truly associated with difference in fetal gender. Supporters of this belief suggest that it might have something to do with testosterone, the so-called male hormone that can influence strength and aggression. Men with high levels of testosterone, they say, may produce more sperm that are likely to yield male children.

The belief that strong men are more likely to have male children is the complete opposite of another school of thought that is shared by women who talk about gender influences. The counterargument is that it is not the man but the woman who should be dominant to yield a male child. Proponents of this theory encourage women to do masculine things like watch football or wear male clothing in order to have a boy.

This line of thinking has its own set of studies in support. An American author in the late nineteenth century looked at birth records for children born in the city versus those in more rural settings.[10] He demonstrated higher ratios of males to females for children born in the country. He reasoned that women in the country do more physical labor and are therefore stronger and more likely to produce boys.

Another study looked at the biographies of all the women in a "Who's Who" type of publication that included women who were successful in their fields over a forty-year timespan.[11] For each woman listed, the researchers noted whether she had children and how many were boys. Among the women who had children, there were 221 sons and 156 daughters, yielding a markedly different ratio from what would be expected by chance. The authors suggested that successful women may have more dominant characteristics that lead to a more hospitable environment for male babies. Regardless of which one of these opposing viewpoints has merit, small differences in sex ratio are unlikely to have much effect on one individual's efforts to influence her baby's sex. So if a woman wants to wear a football jersey to bed, it is still far from a safe bet that she will conceive a boy that night.

Modern science teaches us that the sex of a baby is not determined by any particular quality of either parent, but rather by the particular type of sperm cell that happens to fertilize the female egg. Sperm cells that carry an X chromosome will produce a female embryo, and sperm cells with a Y chromosome will produce a male. With this in mind, modern theorists have entertained different explanations for the sex ratios described by population scientists. Perhaps there are particular qualities of the father that favor a production of one type of sperm over another. Or perhaps there are qualities of the mother that make the egg more receptive to one or the other type of sperm cell. Trying to find differences between the X- and Y-bearing sperm cells, researchers have looked for differences that might explain how one type might behave differently from another.

One difference that has been described is a slight difference in the lifespan between these types of sperm cell. The X chromosome sperm do not survive quite as long, so that the supply of these cells may be more quickly depleted when there is a high demand for sperm production. In support of this idea, there may be a higher proportion of male infants (that is, those arising from the Y-bearing sperm) when men have sex more often, since that would use up the X-bearing sperm more quickly. An article examining sex ratios in successive years of marriage supported this theory.[12] It showed that more males are conceived during the first year after marriage or in recently reunited couples than in later years of marriage. Supposedly this is due to newlyweds being more sexually active, and it is during the first year of married life that the frequency of sexual intercourse is at its peak.[13] Another researcher measured the proportion of X-bearing sperm in men who abstained from sex compared with those who had frequent ejaculation.[14] This study showed that there was a slightly increased number of X-bearing sperm in the ejaculate of men who had held off from any ejaculation for at least four days. However, the difference was not considered great enough to affect the sex ratio. Even if subtle differences exist in the proportion of Y-bearing sperm in one sperm sample versus another, it is unlikely that a couple could use this fact to reliably produce offspring of a desired gender.

Another very popular old remedy for producing a baby of a particular gender has to do with the timing of intercourse relative to the woman's ovulation. Depending on which authority one listens to, a boy is more likely to be conceived only on certain days of the month. This idea is a pervasive one that has been voiced in various cultures and in historical times that came long before there was any idea that ovulation occurred in the middle of the menstrual cycle, or even that there was such a thing as ovulation at all.[15] For example, the Susruta Samhita, a medical text compiled in India in second century CE, instructs couples desiring a boy to engage in intercourse only on even days in the first half of a woman's menstrual cycle, while a daughter could be conceived only on odd days. The Ishimpo, a collection of ancient Chinese works collected between the seventh and tenth centuries CE, prescribes a similar regimen, but the male results from intercourse during the first three days following menses, and a female during the next two days. Avicenna, the noted eleventh-century Persian physician, also divided the postmenstrual phase based on gender, but he allowed five days for conception of sons and four more for daughters. As we now know, the most fertile time in a woman's menstrual cycle is when she ovulates, about two weeks after the beginning of her period. So presumably these ancient Chinese and Persians were having sex on other days, too, or their efforts to bear sons would have resulted in very few children indeed.

The version of this recipe that has remained popular in present-day chat rooms actually states the opposite: that girls are more likely to be conceived early in the menstrual cycle, while boys are conceived closer to the time of ovulation. Proponents of this theory point to some data that Y-bearing sperm (the ones that will become boys) tend to be slightly lighter and move faster than X-bearing sperm. Therefore, having sex very close to the time of ovulation should increase the number of Y-bearing sperm that reach the egg. Slower moving X-bearing sperm are more likely to reach the egg when they are deposited a few days before ovulation. So this theory suggests that couples who want to have daughters should have sex a few days before ovulation occurs, so those lumbering X chromosome sperm cells will have time to get to the party.

This idea may sound reasonable, but science has shown that there is no truth to it. One study asked women to give daily urine and blood samples so that researchers would know exactly which day they ovulated, and also had them keep a diary of exactly which days they had sex.[16] The results proved that the number of boys and girls was the same regardless of whether the couple had sex before, during, or after ovulation. Another study looked at women who got pregnant while using "natural family planning," a technique of timing efforts to get pregnant (or to avoid conception) based on natural changes that a woman may notice in her body at the time of ovulation.[17] With ovulation measured by shifts in body temperature and changes in cervical mucus production, the author examined the resulting gender of babies born after sex around that time. This study showed a slightly *lower* proportion of boys born after sex occurred during the most fertile days. This result goes against the idea that the boys-to-be sperm are faster. Regardless, these studies suggest that couples are not able to control the sex of their offspring just by deciding when to have sex.

Controlling gender by "timing of intercourse" may not refer only to when sex happens in relation to ovulation, but also to timing of orgasm. The relevant piece of folklore advice for this issue recommends that a man who wants to have a boy should make sure that his lady love "comes first." A man who climaxes before his partner does, it is said, is bound to have a girl. The origin of this idea is uncertain, but again may be rooted in antiquity.[18] The English translation of Leviticus 12:2 states, "When a woman gives birth and bears a male child. . . ." However some Hebrew scholars translate the phrase "gives birth" as "emits seed." In the Babylonian Talmud, a Rabbi Isaac discusses this passage and draws the conclusion that a woman who has an emission first (i.e., before her husband) will bear a son. Of course, Talmudic scholars had no concept of female ovulation, so the seed that was thought to be emitted would occur during orgasm. So for husbands who desired a male child, those Talmudic scholars advocated for them to hold back on ejaculation until their wives were satisfied.

Such theories may be based on conjecture and loose interpretation, but they sound more reasonable when placed in a scientific framework. Female orgasm does not seem to be related to infant gender, but the increase in vaginal fluid that occurs during arousal does make the vagina more alkaline. The idea that the relative acidity or alkalinity of the vagina could influence the likelihood of conception dates back at least to the 1930s. It was then that a German obstetrician named Unterberger tried to prove that sperm were more likely to survive in an alkaline environment. [19] He instructed women to douche with baking soda prior to having intercourse and was able to demonstrate a high rate of male babies born to these women. He suggested that the higher pH of the vaginal fluid was more conducive to Y-bearing sperm than those carrying the X chromosome. The results were popularized at the time in medical conferences and in the *New York Daily News*, leading proponents to claim that gender could be controlled by precoital douching: with bicarbonate for a boy, and with vinegar for a girl. Unfortunately, later research did not bear out Dr. Unterberger's findings.

In the 1960s, an obstetrician named Landrum Shettles took several of these pieces of gender-predicting advice and synthesized a formula that he assured women could help them choose their baby's sex. [20] Shettles accepted the idea that Y-bearing sperm were faster and that they would swim more vigorously in an alkaline environment. He was also of the opinion that these sperm would die sooner, which ran counter to some of the advice mentioned earlier. Putting all these ideas together, he reasoned that the best chance of conceiving a male would occur if semen were ejaculated as close as possible to the egg, as soon as possible after the egg ovulated, and with the highest possible pH. The "Shettles method," as it became popularly known, involved several steps that made these characteristics possible. To conceive a boy, a couple should have sex on the day of ovulation following a baking soda douche for the woman and a several-day period of abstinence for the male.

Furthermore, sex should take place in a rear entry position with the man depositing semen as deeply as possible in the vaginal canal and only after the woman has reached orgasm. For a girl, the opposite would be the case: sex before ovulation in a face-to-face position with shallow penetration, following a vinegar douche by the woman and frequent prior ejaculation by the man. For couples who took the pains to follow all of these steps, Shettles claimed an 85 percent success rate in having a child of the desired sex.

Shettles's book was popular enough that it attracted the attention of a number of researchers who wanted to see if he was right. Unfortunately, no one else was able to match his rates of success. An Australian study recruited couples who were motivated enough to get a child of the desired gender that they were willing to strictly adhere to this method.[21] Despite going through all these steps, these couples had babies with the desired gender at a rate no better than chance through seventy-three pregnancies over four years. A larger study involving 185 couples found that only 39 percent had a baby of the desired sex, although this study left out the douching requirement.[22] Even though Shettles wrote his book fifty years ago, his method is still talked about on some pregnancy advice websites. Adherents of his method say it definitely worked for them, and the poor success that others had was only due to failing to follow the instructions exactly. Even if any individual component of the Shettles method were scientifically verified (which they are not), it would be impractical for a couple to be so regimented and restricted in their lovemaking for what may be months while trying to conceive a child. It would probably be better to let them enjoy sex however they want it, without worrying about the smell of vinegar or the loss of face-to-face intimacy.

Yet another school of thought on how to conceive a child of a particular gender involves the role of diet. Folklore in various cultures recommends the ingestion of male genital organs, from various animals and in various forms, to get a male child. The reason why a primitive culture would embrace such a suggestion seems obvious; it is another example of the like-breeds-like thinking that is often seen in folkloric advice. In modern society, however, the concept of eating ground testicles or dried foreskin will probably not sell that well no matter how much a woman wants to conceive a son. One Japanese recommendation urges the mother to consume root vegetables such as turnips and carrots to have a boy; here the food sounds a little more appetizing, since most people would rather eat food that only looks like a penis rather than something made of the real thing.

If phallic foods seem to be the best dietary aids for conceiving a boy, the most common theme in folklore for having a girl would be to have more sweets. Since girls are traditionally known as being sweeter than boys (e.g., made of sugar, spice, everything nice, etc.), some people have thought that this could be due to what a mom eats before pregnancy. Following this principle, a diet rich in sweets and sugars would be more likely to yield a daughter. While there are few mothers who would turn down the idea of having a few extra chocolates or cookies for the sake of their gender selection, it is not reasonable to think that this will actually carry much influence on a baby's gender. Interestingly, though, there is at least one study that supports the notion. In a study of mice that were fed a diet high in carbohydrates and low in fats, their litters included a surprisingly high number of female pups.[23]

Most studies of mammalian species have not shown this to be the case. In fact, there is a good amount of evidence that animals who reproduce in environments where food is plentiful tend to have more male offspring.[24] This theory, known as the Trivers-Willard hypothesis, states that reproduction favors the sex that is most likely to pass on genes to the next generation. So when food is plentiful and a mother is well-fed, she is likely to have more sons, who will be strong and healthy and pass on a lot of their genes. When food is scarce and the mother is undernourished, she is more likely to have daughters, because among scrawny and weak animals, the females are more likely to still attract a mate and reproduce than the males. As unfair and sexist as this sounds, there is a good amount of evidence that bears out this hypothesis for many species of animals.

There is still considerable uncertainty about whether it would hold true for humans. A set of British researchers aimed to find out by examining the diets of 740 British women attending a prenatal clinic.[25] At their first visit, before there was any chance they would know if they were having a boy or a girl, the women gave a detailed report about everything they were eating in the months around conception. The study showed that more boys were born to women who ate diets with the highest number of calories, and the lowest percentage of boys was born to women who ate the least. The authors also looked at individual foods in the diets of these mothers and found that the only food more likely to be consumed by mothers of boys was breakfast cereal. There was nothing in particular about breakfast cereal that was thought to influence gender, but the authors remarked that it might just be a marker for having breakfast and therefore a healthy diet of three square meals a day. So it is unlikely that an extra bowl of Wheaties will significantly improve a woman's odds of having a son, but she may want to make sure she is getting an adequate number of calories each day.

If the old sayings favor sugar and spice for girls, one might think the opposite holds true for boys. Indeed, there are several recommendations that suggest that salty and savory foods are the ones that may yield more sons. The scientific way to look at this proposal would be to suggest that a salty diet would be richer in minerals like sodium and potassium. The British study just mentioned did show such an effect, with the sex ratio favoring boys in the women who consumed the most sodium and potassium. A more dramatic effect was shown by a German doctor in the 1930s who experimented with marine worms.[26] He showed that by manipulating the water in which these worms grew to be more or less salty, he could change the sex ratio of the baby worms that were born. Even if he could accurately tell the sex of a baby worm, it is a big stretch to think that this same principle could apply to humans.

The idea was refined and popularized in a book titled *The Preconception Gender Diet* that was published in 1982.[27] This book claimed that a diet rich in certain minerals including sodium would increase the chance of having a boy. The writers based their recommendations on a study that examined the effect of a specific diet administered to both women and their partners in the four to six weeks prior to attempts at conception.[28] For couples who wanted boys, the researchers prescribed a diet high in salt and potassium and provided additional potassium supplement tablets. Couples trying to have girls were given a diet that was low in salt and potassium and high in calcium, with an extra calcium and vitamin D tablet daily. In this study, 80 percent of couples produced a child of the gender that they were trying for. Unfortunately, subsequent studies have not borne out these results. [29] However, one study that involved checking the blood concentrations of these minerals in women trying to get pregnant showed that lower levels of sodium and higher levels of calcium predicted a higher chance of having a girl.[30]

Still, there is not much evidence that loading up on salty snacks before pregnancy is going to increase the chance of having a boy. But unless a woman already has problems with blood pressure or swelling, it probably isn't going to hurt.

Despite the number and variety of recommendations for choosing the sex of one's child, there does not seem to be any surefire way to have any control over the situation. Even in countries where male babies are more valued, there hasn't been any shift in the sex ratio due to people who follow such advice. Of course, there are always people who will claim that the method in question is successful, since it will work half the time. So there will continue to be advocates on the Internet who swear that a particular diet or sex position or article of clothing can really help you to conceive a girl. But even if evidence suggests that we can budge the sex ratio for a whole population a little bit one way or the other by adopting certain behaviors, it is unlikely that a particular couple will be able to reliably choose their baby's gender just by following one of these pieces of advice. The best advice remains for couples to take what nature gives them and love their baby no matter what the gender.

4

GENDER PREDICTION

It may not be possible for a couple to manipulate the forces of nature enough to engineer a boy or a girl, but that doesn't stop anyone from spending the next nine months trying to figure out what they are going to have. It seems like no characteristic invites as much speculation as the baby's gender. Sure, there might be some discussion about whether the baby will look like Mom or Dad. And occasionally some parents may wonder about things like hair color, or length, or eye color. But none of those come close to the endless speculation on whether the baby will be male or female. The first question that is always asked in the delivery room (if the answer is not already known) is not "Does my baby look okay?" or even "Is my baby healthy?" The first announcement that the delivering attendant is expected to make is "It's a [gender of baby]!"

In some cultures, this may be because of the importance placed on the gender, usually with boys valued higher because of the patriarchal nature of those societies. More modern practitioners of the "guess the gender" game say it is for more practical purposes: what color to paint the nursery, for example, or what gifts to ask for at the baby shower. More often than not, gender prediction is just a source of amusement for the expectant mother, her family, and her friends. Everyone likes to play games of chance, and what better chance can a person get than with a game where the odds of winning are fifty–fifty? Half of the family and friends playing along will be able to gloat about being right, so of course they will continue to pass on whatever pieces of folklore they use to make their predictions. For all of these reasons, there have been quite a number of methods passed along from one generation to the next about predicting what sex the infant will be.

Many predictions are based on activities that have two outcomes, just because there are two genders. A widespread recommendation is to suspend a chain over the pregnant woman's abdomen (some say with her wedding ring attached) to see which way it will swing. Sources vary as to whether it is meaningful to have it swing in a line versus in a circle. Whether the distinction is back and forth, up and down, or clockwise and counterclockwise, the premise is always that it has to be one thing or another. So it is not surprising that once again, right and left frequently come into play.

As described in the previous chapter, the right side of the body has long been associated with greater heat and strength, and therefore with being more male. So there are many folkloric suggestions that changes on the right side of the body signal a boy baby. The idea dates back to the ancient writings of Hippocrates, who wrote that the male fetus lies on the right side of the womb, while the female lies on the left. For some people the prediction is simply that a mom's belly that is more tilted to the right is carrying a boy. For others, the distinctions are more subtle. The medieval physician Albertus Magnus described other right-sided changes that occur in the woman carrying a boy. According to him, a woman's right eye is brighter than her left if she is with male child, and her right breast would be bigger than the left. For a girl, the opposite would be true: the left eye is brighter and the left breast bigger.[1]

Similar descriptions exist in other cultures as well, even though their members probably never heard of Hippocrates. For example, women in the Philippines voice the same observation—that a pregnant abdomen that bulges more to the right signifies a boy. In China, it is the pulse that may determine the gender, with a stronger pulse on the right side predicting a boy. There is no scientific evidence to support these theories, perhaps because it would be very hard to objectively measure how bright a woman's eyes are shining or how different the strength of her pulses are.

Internet proponents of the right–left theory frequently cite a particular medical study on this topic. The theory is known as Ramzi's theory, named after Dr. Saad Ramzi Ismail, who wrote a paper that appears on the Internet. The fact that he chose to publish on an Internet site, and not in a medical journal where research has to be evaluated by one's peers, immediately casts doubt over his findings. Nevertheless, he claims to have accurately predicted fetal gender with 97 percent accuracy by performing transvaginal ultrasounds on over five thousand women over a ten-year time span.[2] By performing these ultrasounds very early in pregnancy (around six weeks of gestation), he could see which side of the uterus the placenta began to grow on. He observed that 97.2 percent of male fetuses had a placenta on the right side of the uterus, and 97.5 percent of female fetuses had a placenta growing on the left. A more modest study appears in an Iranian journal that looks at early sonograms in two hundred pregnant women.[3] These researchers did not find as great a difference in right versus left placentas, but claimed that 73 percent of female fetuses had a placenta growing on the front wall of the uterus, as opposed to just 27 percent of male fetuses. No good explanations have been proposed for why gender should have anything to do with the side of the uterus where the placenta attaches. But if these studies are to be taken at face value, then perhaps additional testing is warranted.

Another common characteristic that women claim will provide a hint at the baby's gender is the level of activity. Boys are often perceived to be more active and play rough, while girls are encouraged to be more docile and gentle. It follows, then, that this must be the way babies behave even before they are born. Does your baby kick you endlessly in the ribs from morning to night? Well, that must be a boy. Feeling little delicate movements? Only a girl would move that way. Although these comments are heard frequently today, they have a much older origin. The Roman physician Soranus suggested that male fetuses have more acute and vehement movements, while female movements tend to be slower and more sluggish.[4] Other cultures also feature this folklore, with writings from Egypt and the Far East claiming that boys kick harder, and mothers perceive them as being more active.[5]

Of course, fetal movement is influenced by many factors other than gender. Sometimes a placenta that is located in front of the uterus can act like a cushion that makes pregnant women perceive less movement. The amount of amniotic fluid that is present can also change the perception of movement, since a lot of fluid will give babies plenty of room to stretch. Gestational age plays a big role, with movement first felt around twenty weeks and then increasing from there. By thirty weeks, the number of fetal leg movements in one minute reaches a maximum. As the pregnancy gets closer to the due date, this number tends to decrease as the space available for those big kicks is reduced. In one study, fetal leg movements were studied by videotaping ultrasounds on a group of women who were examined at regular intervals at the end of pregnancy, as well as videotaping the infants' behavior after birth.[6] In this study, boys displayed more leg movements per minute than girls both inside and outside the womb. Although it is not possible to assign gender based on any specific number of kicks, it appears that there may be some truth to this particular observation.

Some gender prediction tales do not deal with the baby's movement, but rather how the baby is resting. Most commonly, one hears predictions based on whether the woman appears to be carrying the baby high in her belly or low. Cultures differ on what is the significance of each. In ancient Egypt and modern-day Taiwan,[7] carrying low was thought to signify a boy, while cultures in central and western Asia associate girls with carrying low.[8] A study of women in Baltimore set out to settle this argument.[9] One hundred and four women who did not know the sex of their baby were asked what sex they thought it was and why they thought so. Thirty percent thought that the way they carried the baby had something to do with the gender. The participants were asked whether they felt that they carried their babies "all up front" or spread lower, and abdominal shape was also rated by an independent observer. Neither the woman's perception of her shape nor that of the independent observer could predict the gender of the baby within. Interestingly, women were split down the middle as to which gender they thought they carried when they felt they were carrying high.

There was one significant observation that came out of this study. Women who had more than twelve years of education correctly predicted the gender of their baby more often than less educated women. When asked for the basis for these predictions, women more commonly cited dreams or feelings rather than issues related to abdominal shape. It's hard to say why a more educated woman would have more accurate dreams; gender prediction is not generally something taught in schools! Two other studies, one from China[10] and one from Alabama,[11] also demonstrate that women are most likely to predict fetal gender based on intuition or hunches rather than other folkloric determinants. Unfortunately, neither of these studies actually kept track of the baby's sex at birth, so they do not offer any insight into how often these hunches are correct.

In one study that did keep track, women who did not know what they were having were asked if they had a strong intuitive feeling about their baby's gender.[12] They all gave their opinion just about seven months into the pregnancy. A little over half of the women reported a strong hunch about the sex, but their chance of being correct was still no better than chance. Of note, about two-thirds of the women thought they would have a boy. This study would suggest that no matter how educated a woman is, she is not likely to be able to tell fetal gender by intuition alone.

One of the most ancient sources of information about pregnancy in general, and fetal gender in particular, is the pregnant woman's urine. Nowadays women associate urine testing with pregnancy because they are asked to give a sample at every prenatal visit. Way before there were prenatal appointments, caregivers looked at urine as an easily available source of information about pregnancy. One of the oldest medical writings in existence mentions its use. The Berlin papyrus is an ancient Egyptian document thought to have been written around 1350 BCE. It contains a description of diagnosing pregnancy by having a woman urinate on a collection of barley and wheat grains.[13] If both grains sprouted, then that was a sign that the woman was pregnant. This line of thought harkens back to the association between fertility and seeds, with growth being a literal and symbolic sign of fertility. The reason that two different kinds of grain was recommended, though, was to gain some insight into the baby's gender. If the barley sprouted first, the child would be male; a girl would result if the wheat sprouted first.

There are not too many medical studies that cite ancient papyrus documents as the inspiration for research. Nevertheless, this antiquated notion seems to have captured the fancy of some scientific types.[14] A German researcher in 1933 used urine that was diluted and aerated with filter paper to see if it promoted growth of these grains. He found that when the barley grew more quickly, it predicted a girl in 80 percent of the cases. The test was repeated in 1962, this time with samples from forty pregnant women, with a few samples of urine from men and nonpregnant women to act as controls. They also used not two but four different kinds of grain, with various degrees of urine dilution to make sure they were covering all bases. They found that nothing grew with the control urine, but there was at least some growth in twenty-eight out of the forty pregnant samples. They theorized that pregnant urine contains high amounts of hormones excreted as waste that may serve to act as fertilizer, or at least to overcome the other ingredients in urine that might suppress growth. So those ancient Egyptians were onto something in devising the very first urine pregnancy test.

However, the order in which the grains sprouted did not predict gender any better than chance. The discrepancy between their findings and those mentioned previously may be a matter of semantics. They point out that the translation of the ancient Egyptian terms is not agreed on by different sources. Although one English translation uses the term "wheat" for the boy-grain and "spelt" for the girl-grain, a German translation uses "barley" to describe the grain for boys and "buckwheat" as the grain for girls. The German translator pointed out that the word for barley in German has a feminine gender, while the German word for wheat is masculine, but the words in Egyptian have an opposite association. In English, we don't assign genders to our nouns, so these subtleties may not seem relevant. As confusing as all the terminology is, it seems safe to conclude that whatever grain you want to call it, it is not that helpful in telling what gender a baby will be.

Most women do not have a readily available supply of cereal seeds to test their urine with, even if it were helpful. Instead, they may look for other more common household items that may be used for gender prediction. The most common urine test recommended on various Internet sites is the Drano test. According to its proponents, mixing a pregnant woman's urine with the bathroom solvent Drano can predict fetal gender, with a green hue indicating a male fetus and an amber or brownish tint indicating female. The origin of this idea is obscure. Drano was invented in 1923, so this recommendation cannot have existed for too long. Yet it was so well publicized by 1982 that a physician in Wyoming tested the theory on his own patients and published the results in the *Journal of the American Medical Association*.[15] He found that the chance of correctly predicting a boy from the test was no better than flipping a coin. A pair of Canadian doctors performed a similar study fifteen years later.[16] They remarked that, although the first study used green to indicate male and brown to indicate female, they had heard from patients that the opposite was true. So they made their calculations both ways and still found that gender could not be predicted no matter what color you called the Drano-urine mixture. A phone call to the SC Johnson company, the manufacturer of Drano, yielded no insight as to the idea's origin. However, the company has an official statement discouraging the use of its product for gender prediction. That is probably wise, since Drano is a highly caustic substance; even if there were a shred of truth to the notion, it is not worth risking a chemical burn or inhaling toxic fumes to get some insight into the gender of your baby.

An extremely popular gender selection technique that avoids the mess of urine and the danger of bathroom solvents is simply consulting a chart. With the explosion of websites devoted to pregnancy and pregnancy folklore, the recommendation to consult a gender prediction chart is heard more and more. The most commonly cited chart is the "ancient" Chinese calendar method. Many websites post some variation of a table that plots age along one axis and month of the year along another axis. Match up a woman's age at the time of conception with the month when she conceived and, voila: the corresponding box will tell you if you should expect a girl or a boy. Of course, there is a lot of wiggle room to excuse false predictions, since it is common for a woman to be not *exactly* sure of the time of conception, and the Chinese calendar uses lunar months that do not line up with the Western month names that are listed on the tables. Websites touting this technique make it sound very reliable and authoritative, since it is invariably said to have been discovered within a royal tomb outside of Beijing seven hundred years ago. These sites also repeat the fact that the scrolls in which the table originated are housed in the "Institute of Science" in Beijing. Since typing this name into various search engines does not identify any such institution, and a search of Chinese science museum websites does not include these scrolls, the whole account smacks of fabrication and fancy. Most of the websites reproduce the same table, but there are some that have the gender listed in a different order, further calling into question the subject's authenticity.

For whatever reason, people are convinced that ancient civilizations had answers to questions that we have somehow lost. The Mayan civilization is known for its attention to dates and numbers, with some people believing that the Mayans could predict natural disasters and even the end of the world with their calendar system. So of course, they should be able to predict gender with a calendar. The technique found on the Internet for using a Mayan calendar to predict gender, and the accompanying mumbo jumbo, are fairly similar to the one that comes from the ancient Chinese. As flimsy and transparent as these websites appear, there has been some attempt to scientifically prove their accuracy. A study of two calendars (the Chinese Gender Calendar and the Georgian Prediction System) found an accuracy rate for both of about 50 percent among 370 racially diverse babies.[17] The 50 percent rate was also confirmed in a study where the researchers specifically converted calendar dates into a Chinese lunar calendar.[18] As expected, consulting a gender prediction chart is no better at predicting gender than flipping a coin.

Another way that women are supposed to know the sex of the baby they are carrying is by listening to their stomachs. Specifically, the amount of nausea that a woman experiences during her pregnancy is said to be related to the baby's gender. Daughters, according to folklore, will make their mothers particularly queasy, while sons will not have quite as much of a nausea-inducing effect. This effect was first noted by the ancient Greek physician Hippocrates, who in his book *Aphorisms* noted that women carrying a daughter appear pale, while women carrying sons appear ruddy and well-fed. Some have speculated that girls are by nature more finicky about food, and so they cause their mothers to eat less while they are pregnant. Perhaps the observation is just passed on to make nauseous women feel better about going through all the discomfort, at least the ones who are looking forward to having a girl.

Maybe the reason it has been passed on is because there is some truth to this observation. Looking at a database of all the pregnancies in Sweden over an eight-year period, a group of researchers observed the sex ratio for women who had to be hospitalized due to severe nausea.[19] Whereas the overall percentage of girls born in Sweden during that time was 48.6 percent, the percentage among women who were admitted to the hospital for severe nausea was 55.7 percent. A study examining the population of Washington State had similar findings.[20] Women who had to be hospitalized in the first three months of pregnancy for severe nausea were 50 percent more likely to have a girl than other women. If the woman was so sick that she had to stay in the hospital for three days or more, she had an 80 percent increased chance of delivering a daughter! The reason for this effect is uncertain, but it is thought to be due to differences in hormone levels between mothers carrying daughters and those carrying sons. Some have suggested that it is the fetal sex that influences the secretion of certain hormones; others maintain that the preexisting hormonal environment of the mother influences which sex is conceived or takes hold. Either way, a woman who is looking green around the gills may expect more pink in the nursery.

The flipside to girls causing nausea is that boys may cause an increased appetite. Craving more food is said to be a sign of having a boy. It is well known that boys, on average, weigh more than girls at birth. This leads some to believe that, in order to put on that extra weight, the boy fetus needs more nourishment. Therefore, he will make the mother hungrier so that she will eat more and provide that extra weight. Actually, the difference in average birth weights between boys and girls is only about three ounces, so there would not have to be a whole lot of extra intake. But some still use this as an excuse to eat a little more.

A group of researchers in Boston evaluated this idea a bit more closely.[21] They administered a detailed questionnaire to 402 women in the second trimester to find out exactly what they were eating. They found that women carrying a boy consumed on average 10 percent more calories than women carrying girls. Unfortunately, the study does not specify how many of these women already knew the sex of their baby, so this may have been a psychological effect. Still, it is interesting to note that despite this difference, there was no difference in the mother's weight gain between the two groups. It may be that the women carrying male fetuses had a metabolism that was revved up a bit higher, allowing them to eat more without gaining weight. The authors propose that this may be an effect of male hormones made by the fetal testicle. Although none of these studies show effects dramatic enough to make an accurate prediction for most women, there does appear to be some evidence that women can get a better idea of what sex the baby will be judging by their appetite.

Of all the gender prediction techniques that are talked about, perhaps none has received as much attention from patients and doctors alike as the fetal heart rate. Based on personal experience, hardly a week goes by without a prospective parent asking whether the heart rate at a prenatal visit indicates a girl or a boy. The normal fetal heart rate varies between 120 and 160 beats per minute. A baseline over 140, so the saying goes, indicates a female fetus, while a lower baseline predicts a boy.

It is unclear where this idea originated, but it cannot have ancient origins like many other pieces of folklore. In fact, the first time that anyone was able to listen to human fetal heart tones through the abdominal wall occurred in 1822, so the idea could only have arisen in the last two hundred years. It is possible that the theory started out based on what has been seen in other species. For candlers (that is, farmers who hold a chicken egg up to the light to see if there is a baby chick within), female chick embryo hearts are seen to beat faster than males in the final days of incubation.[22] Perhaps farmers in earlier times made this observation and applied it to human fetuses.

By 1887, however, the idea was already a matter of debate. The obstetrician Charpentier wrote a textbook about pregnancy in that year, and said that conversation about whether fetal heart rate could predict gender had started "in recent years."[23] He mentioned that two colleagues of that era had done studies that proved a faster heartbeat in female fetuses, but he also cited two other contemporaries who showed that there was no such relationship.

For whatever reason, once the idea took hold, it persisted in the public imagination. Perhaps this notion is repeated because it seems plausible and scientific. Maybe it's because (unlike other notions about degree of nausea or eye brightness) heart rate is something that is measurable and objective. Because it is a theory that can be tested, scientists keep returning to the question repeatedly, even though the results are consistent in showing that there is not really any difference between male and female fetuses.

Early studies that were done used stethoscopes to listen to the baby's heart rate through the abdominal wall in various stages of pregnancy.[24] Speculating that these studies showed no difference because a stethoscope may not be the most exact way to measure, researchers have conducted more recent studies that use either Doppler monitors (the electronic monitors that most modern doctors use in their offices)[25] or ultrasound measurements.[26] Again, neither of these techniques of measurement proved any more successful at proving a difference.

Fetal heart rates are known to get lower over the course of pregnancy. Small fetuses have more rapid heart rates than large fetuses, just like children have faster heart rates than adults. So perhaps this difference between boys and girls is only present at the beginning of pregnancy? Not at all, based on a study of women who had undergone in vitro fertilization.[27] In these pregnancies, transvaginal ultrasounds are done routinely from a very early point in pregnancy, as soon as a heart rate can be measured. The study failed to show any difference, even in these tiniest of pregnancies. Maybe there is variation over other times during gestation? No, according to another study that calculated an average rate for each fetus over multiple prenatal visits that occurred from the beginning to the end of pregnancy.

How about if you compare siblings? Perhaps the difference in heart rates is a "relative" thing. One study compared heart rate monitors in forty-one families where the parents had one child of each sex.[28] The authors hoped to show that, even if the absolute number of beats per minute was not different, the boys might always have had a lower number than their sisters. Unfortunately, the answer was again no, with no pattern of differences detected. The evidence certainly seems to stack up that there is really no difference between boys and girls in this respect.

In one of the few studies where there was a meaningful difference, fetal heart rate tracings were compared in the final hour before birth.[29] The study looked at the tracings that are used on the labor floor for women in labor to check on the baby's well-being during the labor process. In the final stages of labor, female fetuses were noted to have significantly higher baseline heart rates than males. The difference was not seen earlier in labor, but the researchers pointed out that the difference held true even after taking other variables into account such as gestational age, length of labor, and type of pain relief. So there may actually be some effect of gender on fetal heart rate as a baby prepares for birth. Unfortunately, that is unlikely to help the couple trying to predict whether to paint the nursery blue, since they will at that point be less than an hour away from welcoming their newborn in person.

Even with all the scientific evidence against it, the idea of girls having faster heart rates lives on. It may be the most frequently encountered bit of folklore that prenatal caregivers encounter in everyday practice. No doubt this myth persists for the same reason that many of these bits of folkore do: because no matter how crazy the reasoning, the gender prediction techniques will always be right half the time. No amount of research or evidence is going to stop these notions from being passed along, since one out of two people will swear that they work.

Perhaps one of the soundest pieces of advice about predicting gender came from the eighteenth-century French obstetrician Francois Mauriceau. He instructed his colleagues to ask their patients what sex of baby they were most hoping for. Whatever they tell you, he said, predict that their baby is of the opposite gender. If the doctor is right, he will seem a genius. And if he is wrong, according to Mauriceau, the couple will be so happy that they will not care or remember what the doctor thought. This recommendation sounds at least as accurate as any of the old wives' tales that have been discussed.

5

FOOD AVERSIONS AND CRAVINGS

Once a woman shares the news of her pregnancy, there is no shortage of recommendations about what to eat and drink. Friends and relatives are eager to share advice about "eating for two" and what kind of diet makes the healthiest pregnancy. In terms of advice on being healthy, there is not much difference between what a woman hears from her caregiver and what she hears from her older relatives. Everyone agrees that a woman should maintain a healthy diet while expecting, and that she should avoid substances known to be harmful, like alcohol or recreational drugs. Both camps will usually give advice about eating fruits and vegetables and being careful not to overdo it on the sweets. It would seem that a lot of advice about diet in pregnancy is in the mainstream and not dismissed as folklore.

Where the old wives differ from mainstream medicine is in the notion that what a woman eats during pregnancy is not always completely under her control. Rather, her diet is often subject to the whims and fancies of the baby itself. Many cultures and social groups express the opinion that babies cause all sorts of changes in their mothers' tastes and appetites, and these changes are what drive her choices of what to eat. Issues like nausea, aversions, and cravings are common in pregnancy, and the explanations for them and the effects that they have are the subject of many old wives' tales.

At the beginning of pregnancy, diet is often restricted by nausea. Nausea is such a common symptom of early pregnancy that many women cite this as the reason that they suspect they are pregnant in the first place. The combination of missing a period and suddenly having one's stomach turned by certain smells or food sightings is a certain sign of pregnancy, or so the saying goes. In fact, nausea and vomiting are extremely common symptoms, experienced by 70 to 85 percent of pregnant women. The first descriptions of morning sickness appear in Egyptian papyrus documents from 2000 BCE, and Hippocrates mentions it as a sign of pregnancy in his *Aphorisms*.

As unpleasant as this sensation is for the expectant mother, she is often consoled by the fact that it means she will have a healthy pregnancy. Nausea is often called a "good" sign, and putting up with all that retching will pay off in having a healthy baby. From ancient times, women have recognized that those who vomit frequently are less likely to miscarry, while women who have no such symptoms may have nonviable or unhealthy pregnancies. One early nineteenth-century physician went so far as to prescribe his pregnant patients ipecac syrup in order to induce vomiting, believing that their pregnancies would be more successful if he could keep the nausea going until the fourth month.[1] Although his intentions were understandable, few women are likely to have been willing to endure more vomiting than their queasy stomachs already produced.

The notion of nausea being a healthy sign, though, is not far from the truth. Women with frequent nausea and vomiting in the first trimester are indeed less likely to miscarry. A systematic review of medical literature about nausea and vomiting in pregnancy confirms that these women are less likely to lose the pregnancy, and it also shows that they are less likely to have children with congenital malformations or are less likely to deliver prematurely.[2]

Why would nausea be protective against these bad pregnancy outcomes? It is probably not so much an effect of the nausea, but rather that the nausea is a result of the same chemical that keeps the pregnancy healthy. The chemical thought to be largely responsible for this symptom is human chorionic gonadotropin (HCG), which is manufactured by the placenta. Healthy placentas that manufacture plenty of HCG and that have good connections to maternal circulation are ones that are likely to do the best job of keeping the fetus healthy and well-perfused. Unfortunately, the high levels that get into the mother's circulation don't make her feel so great.

Other folklore tries to explain why women should have to put up with three months (or more) of queasiness in the first place. Explanations through history have maintained the idea that there is a direct pipeline from the mother's gut to the developing fetus, and the mother will toss her cookies if she eats something that the baby doesn't like or want. Many women find that there are particular foods that will trigger nausea or indigestion, even when such things never troubled them prior to pregnancy. These aversions may be quite specific, such that a woman can no longer eat cottage cheese or green beans for the duration of her pregnancy. The explanation given is generally along the lines that it is the baby who dislikes these things, and so the mother suffers.

Of course, a ten-week-old fetus does not actually have likes and dislikes, and wouldn't have a means at its disposal to provoke maternal vomiting even if it did. However, many modern health care providers theorize that the nausea and aversions of early pregnancy are an evolutionary adaptation to protect developing babies from substances that might be harmful to them.[3] For one thing, the peak of a pregnant woman's nausea tends to occur early in pregnancy, right when all of its organs and limbs are just forming. This is when a fetus is most vulnerable to agents that might cause birth defects, so it would be an important time for nature to prevent the mother from ingesting harmful substances.

Scientists also note that many foods that tend to trigger nausea, like certain vegetables that have a bitter taste or fibrous texture, also contain more plant-based chemicals. Foods that are starchy and sweet, like corn or potatoes, have fewer of these phytochemicals. In fact, the chance of getting morning sickness is lower in societies that rely on corn as a main staple of the diet.[4] Not that green vegetables are necessarily bad. But many toxins and chemicals in nature have a bitter taste, and making a woman more sensitive to similar flavors might prompt her to avoid chemicals that really do have a negative effect. There are many cases of women who develop aversions to cigarette smoke or beer when pregnant, as evidence that changes in taste may be protective. However, this theory does little to explain the woman who cannot stand chicken salad for a full nine months, or why many women continue to smoke in pregnancy with no repercussions on their diet.

The imagined pipeline between mother's stomach and baby's brain is also the source of folklore about how diet can affect the baby's nature.

Many pieces of folkloric advice stem from literal interpretations of food characteristics and infant characteristics. For example, some caution that having a diet that is full of sour tastes will lead to an infant with a sour disposition. A 1983 survey of American women in a Midwestern community listed several beliefs that women had about how diet could affect the baby's behavior.[5] One woman claimed that consuming a large quantity of chicken or eggs would make a child an early riser. Others said that eating prunes could make a baby more wrinkled, and that eating carrots could result in having a redheaded child.

Of course, none of these precautions have been borne out by any scientific evidence. Since they rely on perceptions of word play or associated meanings, there would be no reason to suppose that eating particular foods like prunes or carrots would really change a baby's appearance. There is one food, though, that has merited a little further exploration: chocolate. Along the lines of thinking that sweet foods may lead to sweet babies, some have claimed that eating chocolate in pregnancy can make a woman feel better and lead to a child with a sweeter temperament.[6] A Finnish study surveyed women who had just given birth and asked them how frequently they ate chocolate during the nine months of their pregnancies. Six months later, the women were asked about their babies' disposition and about behaviors like laughing and crying. The babies of mothers who consumed chocolate daily turned out to be more smiley and easily soothed than those whose mothers abstained.

Still, chocolate is not likely to be the direct cause of these babies acting "sweeter." It may be that women who eat sweets are more indulgent, or happier, or less easily stressed, or some other personality trait that might have a more direct effect on how their babies respond. It may also be that they just think their babies are happier, because they are more likely to give positive answers to survey questions. However, there are scientists and chocolate lovers who point to chemicals in chocolate as having all sorts of health benefits and mood-elevating properties in general, so it is still quite possible that there is some beneficial effect of eating chocolate while pregnant. Just don't eat too much, or the result will be a baby that is overweight!

Most of the folklore in this area deals with how things that the mother eats can affect the way that the baby looks. There is one very pervasive piece of folklore, though, that suggests an influence in the opposite direction: that a characteristic of the baby's appearance influences the mother's diet. It seems that women from all walks of life are led to believe by their colleagues that having a baby with a full head of hair will make their heartburn worse. Women may then limit foods that are known to trigger heartburn, like greasy or spicy items, but it is the baby's shaggy hairdo and not the diet that is blamed. Where this particular piece of folklore started is uncertain. Perhaps it originated with Aristotle, who wrote that the peak of a woman's nausea, and ill feelings in general, occurred when the baby started to grow hair.[7] By the seventeenth century, it could be found among the teachings common to midwives, who were told that if a woman had much heartburn, "the child would be hairy."[8] In more recent surveys, it appears high on the list of frequently heard beliefs, and it is commonly heard in delivery rooms today.

On first hearing of this connection, it doesn't seem like there could be any plausible link. There is no way that baby's hair would do anything to irritate the mother's stomach, and we know that heartburn is a very common symptom of pregnancy and is caused by acid reflux that has nothing to do with hair growth. Nevertheless, the comment is heard so frequently that some researchers decided to examine the issue to see if this is really a case where the old wives could be right due to their keen powers of observation.[9] They asked women in the ninth month of pregnancy to rank just how bad they thought their heartburn was. They then asked the women to submit a photograph of their babies after birth, and an independent coder assigned a numerical value to how dense the baby's hair looked. The value for the amount of heartburn was then compared to the value of infant hairiness. The comparison showed that there was indeed a positive correlation between the amount of heartburn and scalp hair, but no association with the baby's gender, the mother's age, her weight, or any other variable that might have affected the relationship.

The surprising result prompted the authors to find some explanation for why these two characteristics are linked. Perhaps, they wrote, the sort of hormones that influence fetal hair growth may also cause some muscle relaxation that would affect the sphincter muscle that separates the stomach from the esophagus. This might account for the increase in acid reflux that would cause heartburn symptoms. However, they also admit that some ethnicities are just more likely to have hairier children, and maybe women belonging to these groups just happen to experience more heartburn. With the small number of women in the study and the lack of ethnic diversity, it is hard to say if the results apply to everyone. Still the study suggests that, in this case, the old wives may be correct.

Between heartburn, nausea, and food aversions, the pregnant stomach is in for some rough times. The flipside of the coin, however, is the wide variety of cravings and foods that women may enjoy in pregnancy. Food cravings are extremely common among pregnant women, experienced by 50 to 90 percent of American women. Although the most commonly craved foods are sweets such as chocolate, cravings may be for salty or spicy foods, or even for healthy and nutritious foods. Sometimes women demand bizarre combinations of foods, such as pickles and ice cream or brownies on pizza, which trigger either looks of disgust or sympathetic nods, depending on who they are shared with. Cravings may also be cultural. In Egypt, cravings for sweets are rare, and in Japan, the most commonly craved food is rice.[10]

Through history, such cravings have been viewed as a sign of the baby's wants or needs. If a mother craves a sweet treat, observers have thought it must be because the baby is hungry for sweets. In fact, many of those involved in the care of pregnant women have written that denying such cravings may cause great harm for the baby. Trotula of Salerno, writing in the twelfth century, warned against speaking of foods in front of a woman that she is not allowed to have because "if she sets her mind on it and it is not given to her, this occasions miscarriage."[11] Denial of cravings was also thought to affect the developing fetus by causing birthmarks or "stains" in the form of the denied object. For example, a strawberry-shaped mark would occur if the woman was not allowed to eat strawberries when desired. A port-wine stain was said to be the result of denying the pregnant woman wine, but the seventeenth-century obstetrician Mauriceau thought women who said this merely did so as a "Pretext to cover their Liquorishness."[12] In an extreme example of satisfying a "fetal" desire, a nineteenth-century husband was said to have bought his wife a carriage and horses because she feared that if her craving for a new coach were not satisfied, her baby would be born with a carriage-shaped mark.[13]

Others have expressed concern that the denial of cravings threatens not the fetus but the very life of the pregnant woman herself. These writers contend that when a woman has an extremely strong craving for a particular food, then going without it could result in severe illness or pregnancy complications. Such a strong threat has given pregnant women the license to indulge in foods that might otherwise be culturally or socially forbidden. For example, kosher laws dictate that Jewish women must not consume foods like pork, and their religion commands that they go without food completely on the holy day of Yom Kippur. With this superstition in mind, though, some rabbis have held that it is okay if a pregnant woman bends the rules and has a little bacon. The Talmud, a compendium of rabbinical commentary, includes a passage in the book of Yoma that approves of feeding a pregnant woman with such a "morbid desire" because ritual laws are set aside in the face of danger to life.[14]

In modern prenatal care, providers have wised up to the fact that the denial of cravings is not likely to have deleterious effects. Even so, some reliable medical sources of advice on the Internet still claim that in some way it is the needs of the fetus that cause the mother to have such cravings. The increased need for sugar, they say, may signal a need for increased calories, or craving salty foods may be a sign that more potassium intake is needed. The bottom line is that cravings for various foods are very common in pregnancy, and it is difficult to prove that they have anything to do with physiological needs. Every pregnant woman requires a certain increase in the number of calories she consumes and the requirement for minerals to keep her healthy. Some research has investigated whether cravings change with fluctuating levels of hormones or nutritional deficits, but no link has been proven. Some scientists have suggested that there may be chemicals in certain foods that women crave that may have a beneficial effect. Though this may be the case with chocolate (as mentioned prior), overall there is no basis for the assumption that cravings are for foods that will benefit the pregnant woman.

The primary cause of cravings is probably more psychological than physiological. Although there is a small increase in caloric requirements during pregnancy, the type and amount of foods craved are generally much more than a woman typically needs to sustain a healthy pregnancy.[15] It is likely that the prevailing culture gives pregnant women a green light to consume foods or combinations of foods that would otherwise be considered indulgent or extravagant. Perhaps some women take advantage of the culture with a few too many brownies or that extra scoop of ice cream. The danger is that women with cravings have an increased tendency for excessive weight gain in pregnancy. Gaining too much weight may be associated with other pregnancy complications like diabetes and having a baby that is oversized and difficult to deliver. The modern take on cravings that is voiced by most pregnancy care providers is that indulgence is okay up to a point, but healthier substitutions may have to be made for some of the more decadent requests, and nothing should be eaten that would threaten a woman's health.

This can be the case with some cravings that cross the line over to substances that have no nutritional value, a condition known as pica. The word "pica" comes from the Latin name for the magpie, a bird with an indiscriminate appetite that will eat anything. The term is used to describe a craving for substances other than food. It has been noted in various cultures and in people of varying ages, but is very commonly noticed in pregnancy. Some pregnant women experience cravings for such bizarre substances as clay, ice, cornstarch, or dirt. The first description of pica in pregnancy was by Aetius of Amida, a sixth-century physician of Byzantium. He noted that such behavior may begin in the second month of pregnancy and may involve acquiring a taste for earth, egg shells, or ashes. [16]

Pica may even involve the bizarre craving for human flesh. Whether this is a true phenomenon or merely folklore is a matter of conjecture. A cautionary tale that appeared in a sixteenth-century text by J. F. Hubrigkt described a woman who wanted only to eat the flesh of a local baker. Her husband gave the baker money in exchange for permission for her to take three bites of his arm. The baker backed out of the agreement after only two bites, and the woman gave birth to triplets, one of whom was stillborn. The story was meant to advance the notion that denial of cravings put the health of the fetus at risk. [17]

Perhaps such stories are told merely for sheer impact on the audience. Another tale of extreme pica has appeared in numerous medical texts through the nineteenth century, involving a woman who craved flesh so badly that she killed her husband and ate him. The reference appeared for the last time in an obstetrical textbook by the well-known pregnancy authority Joseph DeLee as late as 1943. At that point, the author was not quoting the story as medical fact, but just as a crazy, entertaining anecdote. The author seems to say: no matter how outlandish you think your patients' cravings are, they will never top this one.

Cannibalism may be rarely (if ever) encountered, but consuming substances such as clay and starch are still relatively common. The frequency varies greatly between different cultures, with up to 60 percent of women practicing pica in some societies. Even in an underserved Michigan population, pica was mentioned by one-third of the women in one study.[18] These women voiced the opinion that they were motivated to eat clay or starch because of a perceived need either of the baby or of their own bodies. Some thought that these agents could have a cleansing effect, or that they would supply necessary minerals that would help the pregnancy.

Scientists have remained puzzled why women would feel compelled to eat such seemingly unappetizing and unappealing substances. Some have explored the idea that substances like dirt and clay might actually contain minerals that are needed, like iron, zinc, and calcium. Research looking to prove this theory has not shown that pica can improve levels of these minerals in the mother's blood, and giving mineral supplements does not stop these women from craving non-nutritional substances.[19] The one exception is a craving for ice, which has sometimes been shown to be suppressed by giving a woman extra iron. Why this should be is a mystery, since the ice is simply water and does not affect her iron stores. Another theory is that substances like clay and starch may help with symptoms like heartburn, or hunger in those who are undernourished. Neither of these reasons has been shown to hold water either; most instances of pica do not involve having gastrointestinal symptoms or any particular nutritional deficiency. Finally, there is the theory that these substances may line the stomach and prevent infectious bacteria and viruses or toxins in food from invading and harming the mother. Clay and starch are known to bind certain drugs in the stomach and make them harder to absorb, and they also decrease the ability for certain parasites and bacteria to latch on to the stomach lining. Although this seems the most plausible explanation, it still doesn't seem relevant for the average American woman who has an inexplicable hankering for that cup of cornstarch.

Regardless of the reason for consumption, this practice is one that comes more from within than without. There are no old wives who are telling their loved ones to eat clay or dirt. Nevertheless, there remains a wide variety of recommendations directed at women about what to eat and what to avoid. The majority of common folklore in today's society has merged with well-known pointers about medicine and nutrition. Nutritional advice on the Internet is mostly in line with the same things that women hear from their doctors and midwives: be sure to drink plenty of water, eat a healthy amount of fruits and vegetables, and take a multivitamin each day. Everyone is in agreement that smoking and alcohol are toxic to the growing fetus, and harmful substances like these should be avoided. Still, one might hear the occasional direction to avoid sour foods to avoid a grumpy baby or have more carrots to get that ginger-headed child. As long as the rest of the diet is healthy, such advice may all be taken in fun.

6

PRENATAL INFLUENCES

As soon as they find out they are pregnant, many women will run out to the bookstore or surf the Internet looking for advice and information about the dos and don'ts of pregnancy. They want to know what to do, what to eat, and what to drink in order to have the healthiest baby possible. Of course, they also want to know what they shouldn't do. Behind all the good intentions of growing a strong and healthy baby, there are also fears about something going wrong. What if a woman doesn't eat enough? What if she exercises too much? What if she works too hard? Many questions stem from the nagging thoughts that not doing the right things might somehow endanger the baby's health. Women fear that by not following the rules, they might miscarry or cause the baby harm or to develop abnormally.

Unfortunately, bad things can happen. Women do sometimes miscarry, or have babies born with birth defects. Occasionally, there are particular behaviors that are likely to be the cause, like drinking too much alcohol or taking certain drugs. Most bad outcomes, though, occur at random and are completely unrelated to the mother's activities. It can be very hard for a couple to accept that such events are random, and people have a tendency to look for some cause to explain why such a thing would happen. When parents suffer a pregnancy loss or have a child with an unanticipated problem, they want to know why, and more specifically ask, "Why us?" They closely examine the entire arc of the pregnancy, looking for something that they did that may have led to their misfortune. A woman may perceive that some activity she did, a particular food she ate, or even a thought she had was the cause of the baby's injury, even though there was no reason to think so when it happened.

One can only imagine the long list of possible causes that women might come up with over the course of a full nine months. Consequently, if they fix on particular activities that they think are harmful, they are likely to warn others of their dangers, so other women won't have to share in such misfortune. No doubt this explains why there are so many cautions and restrictions that can be found on websites, warning readers what should be avoided to prevent a bad outcome. Looking back through history and at other cultures, it becomes apparent that this is not just an Internet phenomenon. Chastising pregnant women and prohibiting them from doing as they please has been going on throughout recorded history. It seems every social group has a list of harmful foods to steer clear of, or dangerous activities to avoid. Though these recommendations often have questionable merit, women follow them to make sure their babies will be perfect.

Early in pregnancy, a woman may be most concerned about the possibility of a miscarriage and what she can do to avoid it. Miscarriage is a very common occurrence; one out of about five recognized pregnancies don't make it past the first three months. Since it is so common, most women who get pregnant more than three or four times in their lives will have to deal with a miscarriage at some point. The rest no doubt will know of a relative or friend who miscarried. With so many women spending so much time considering all the things that might have contributed to a miscarriage, the list of old wives' tales dealing with miscarriage is quite long.

Many of the folklore ideas and recommendations about this issue are rooted in the idea of how fragile the pregnancy is at first. Many cultures and historical texts compare the beginning of pregnancy to planting, where the seed is sown in fertile soil but then takes some time to take root and become well established. Similarly, the early pregnancy is thought to be attached to the mother at first by bonds that are tenuous and easy to break. A midwife in Victorian England described it like so:

> The vessels connecting the child to the womb are so extremely delicate as to be broken asunder by various accidental causes. . . . So great is the analogy between animal and vegetable bodies that the . . .

child in this state may be compared to a blossom, which is often blighted and destroyed before the fruit is perfectly set.[1]

It is only later in pregnancy that the baby is firmly attached and ready to "hold on." Most of the recommendations to avoid miscarriage deal with avoiding the kind of jostling or strenuous activity that would sever or loosen the baby's fragile attachments. Some of the typical don'ts that women may hear from friends and relatives include no jumping, no strenuous lifting, no driving over bumpy roads, and no rough contact with others.

Interestingly, there is also a related body of folklore about causing abortion. Throughout history there have been women who find themselves pregnant without wanting to be. Sometimes, they have been so unhappy as to look for advice on how to end the pregnancy. Recommendations on terminating a pregnancy take advantage of the idea that the fetus is only loosely attached to the body, so ending a pregnancy would be merely a matter of shaking it loose. Instructions on how to terminate might include activities like jumping from great heights, being thrown in the air, or riding over very bumpy surfaces. While Hippocrates in his oath vowed never to administer any medicine to cause abortion, he did mention in his book *On the Nature of the Child* that a woman interested in causing an abortion could try "leaping with the heels to the buttocks."[2]

The ancient Roman physician Soranus also wrote about how important it is for the pregnancy to be given time to take root. He agreed that exertion in any form might loosen the baby from its fragile perch in the womb. Miscarriage, he felt, could be induced by vigorous exercise, coughing, sneezing, falling down, or leaping. He recommended against any massage of the abdomen, which could tear the developing pregnancy away, or even bathing in early pregnancy, which could render the texture of the body softer and cause the seed to melt away.[3]

This philosophy can be found again in the writings of Francois Mauriceau, the seventeenth-century French obstetrician. He cautioned women that they should rest in bed for the first few days after they suspected they could be pregnant. He believed that any agitation or jolting could lead to miscarriage, so he cautioned pregnant women not to ride in carriages or on horseback. He considered it safe for them to be carried in sedans or litters, provided they could find willing (or more likely paid) participants to carry them around.[4]

In this same chapter, he cautions against any exertions including the raising of arms above the head. So strict is this rule that he forbids women from even adjusting their hats, since this cannot be done without raising the arms. The rationale he provides is that raising the arms will extend and loosen the ligaments of the uterus and could lead to miscarriage or fetal death. Even though our understanding of anatomy and physiology has come a long way in the last three hundred years, women in various cultures still believe that raising their arms up while pregnant will harm the baby. Even in the last fifty years, surveys of women in rural areas of the United States suggest that many still share this belief. A survey of women in rural California found that this was the most common item of folklore mentioned.[5] The women feared that raising their arms would strangle the baby by pulling on the umbilical cord. Of course there is absolutely no connection between the arms and the uterus, and there is no way that this movement would do anything at all to the baby's umbilical cord. Nevertheless, this concern is still heard occasionally by modern obstetricians from patients who have been told this myth by mothers or grandmothers.

Well into the Victorian era, doctors and old wives alike continued to recommend against overactivity by pregnant women. Authors of guides for pregnant women written during this period advised against many activities that today seem tame. Victorian women who were with child were instructed not to engage in any of the following activities: riding a bicycle, lacing a corset tightly, running a sewing machine by foot, keeping late hours, dancing, or other "fashionable amusements." One physician maintained that the most common causes of miscarriage were "taking long walks; riding on horseback; . . . [taking] a long railway journey; overexerting herself, and sitting up late at night." Instead, women were told to get plenty of rest, wear loose fitting clothing, and avoid anything that could be hurtful.[6]

Nowadays, it seems laughable to forbid pregnant women to dance or stay up late. We know that the baby is very well protected in the womb, and it takes a pretty strong force to cause any harm to the developing fetus. Of course, there are activities that do carry enough force to do real damage; signs on roller coasters and thrill rides that warn pregnant women to stay away are absolutely warranted. But there is still a sentiment on the part of many obstetric patients and their partners that the woman should be "protected" from various activities, including work and exercise. Some of the most common questions that a woman may ask at her first prenatal care visit have to do with how much exercise is okay and if she should scale back on her busy work schedule.

So what does science say about the amount of activity that is appropriate? Can exercise actually cause miscarriages? Many studies have looked at these questions and the answers are overall reassuring. A group of Brazilian authors wrote a review of all the articles they could find that pertained to risks of physical activity and exercise in pregnancy.[7] Out of 3,313 studies that had something to do with physical activity and pregnancy, they included 37 studies that looked at pregnancy outcomes well enough to determine if there was some cause and effect. The consensus among these articles is that light to moderate physical activity does not increase the risk of miscarriage. Many studies even demonstrate that staying active is beneficial for the pregnancy. Women who exercise and stay active throughout pregnancy are less likely to develop other pregnancy complications such as diabetes or preeclampsia.

We now know that the most common reason for miscarriages is some type of chromosomal abnormality. Every human being has twenty-three sets of matched pairs of chromosomes, one from the mother and one from the father. With these pairs getting pulled apart every time a sperm or an egg is made, it is not uncommon for a little genetic material to get left behind or get stuck where it doesn't belong. This kind of genetic mismatching occurs at random, though it happens more commonly in embryos formed from mothers with older eggs, which is why miscarriages are more common in women over the age of thirty-five. There is no reason to think that such random occurrences would be influenced by anything the mother does, whether it is exercise, dancing, or horseback riding.

Interestingly, one study looked at activity levels in women with miscarriages where the genetic makeup of the fetus was known.[8] Among a group of 346 miscarriages where each one was analyzed for whether or not it had a normal number of chromosomes, the mothers were asked about how active they had been in the weeks prior. The women who exercised during pregnancy had a lower risk of having miscarried a chromosomally normal pregnancy. The women who did not exercise were more likely to have miscarried a baby with normal chromosomes. In other words, when a pregnancy miscarries due to a genetic problem, no amount of activity will change it. But in those cases where genetics are not to blame, exercise seemed to be protective against pregnancy loss.

These studies support the notion that generally healthy women should be free to exercise and work without fear of affecting the pregnancy. It may be a different story for women who are identified as having a high risk for miscarriage. For example, an epidemiological study of 5,144 pregnant women compared women with or without a history of miscarriages in the past.[9] The authors asked each woman questions about her employment and home activity. Overall, measures of how much each woman exerted herself did not affect the risk of miscarriage. Looking only at those women who had miscarried two or more times, though, the study showed an association between prolonged standing at work and having another miscarriage. This suggests that there are some women with a predisposition to miscarriage, and they have more reason to follow advice about getting more rest or restricting activity. Nevertheless, it is reassuring to know that the vast majority of pregnant women do not endanger their babies by running or dancing, and they are free to engage in whatever "fashionable amusements" they choose.

One such amusement that is frequently a cause of concern to pregnant women is sex during pregnancy. Through the ages, there have been some authors who were all for it, while some naysayers recommended against it. For the ones who advised against it, the reason often given has to do with those "delicate bonds" mentioned earlier. All that jostling and sudden motion of the pelvis is viewed as harmful to the delicate fetus growing in the womb. Some authors advised against it because they just don't see any point in it: if a woman is already pregnant, then what would she possibly have to gain by having sex?

The ancient Romans cautioned against intercourse in the early part of pregnancy, when the "seed" was felt to be at its most fragile, and the violent motions of the pelvis could lead to its being discharged. Fears related to the effect of pregnancy may also be based on cultural interpretations. For example, among certain ethnic groups in Sri Lanka, excessive intercourse in pregnancy is forbidden because it is thought to generate too much heat, which they believe may be harmful for the fetus.[10]

Other ethnic groups, however, say that it's okay, and even recommended, to have sex during pregnancy. The Kaluli of New Guinea think that male semen is necessary to the proper development of the fetus and believe that a man should keep having sex with his pregnant wife to nourish the fetus and promote growth.[11] An anthropological study in Jamaica revealed that women there too feel that sex in pregnancy is beneficial.[12] The sentiment there is that sexual intercourse improves the womb and keeps the birth canal open so that delivery will be easier when the time comes.

Although there were a lot of prudes in the Victorian era who voiced the opinion that sex in pregnancy is harmful, the general consensus among pregnancy advice websites these days is that sex is safe. Doctors and midwives generally agree that having sex during pregnancy will not cause harm as long as there is no other health condition that would make it dangerous. For example, women who carry a high risk of premature labor or bleeding from the placenta or cervix should not be having sex. These conditions are rare, though, and most women do not need to worry about pelvic thrusts causing harm. There isn't really a lot of medical evidence for this opinion, since there have not been head-to-head studies of identical groups of people who did or did not have sex. However, surveys tell us that most couples continue to have sex throughout pregnancy, and they don't report that it is harmful, so it is accepted as safe.

Most people would argue that sex has its own benefits: it encourages bonding and intimacy, it relieves stress, and it feels good. But it is unlikely to have real benefit for the pregnancy per se. However, one interesting phenomenon has been observed that makes it a little more believable that sex early in pregnancy can be good for the baby. Scientists have demonstrated that women who are exposed to proteins in the father's semen are less likely to develop certain pregnancy complications such as preeclampsia and growth disorders.[13] When couples use a condom, or have sex infrequently before getting pregnant, this protective effect is absent. The rationale for this effect is that unprotected sex introduces semen with the man's genetic material into the mother. When her immune system sees that material repeatedly, it is more likely to be recognized as friendly and not stir up an immunological "attack." Since half of the genetic material in the fetus and the placenta comes from the father, this exposure prevents the mother's immune system from attacking the placenta, which may be an underlying cause of these disorders. Although this effect is observed prior to pregnancy, there is some evidence that it may still be beneficial in the early weeks of pregnancy following conception. So the Kaluli of New Guinea may be on the right track.

Keeping track of what activities are safe in pregnancy may be enough to occupy a woman's thoughts, but there have been many old wives across history that say the thoughts themselves may be harmful! Women have been cautioned to be careful about what thoughts enter their minds because having strong or unpleasant emotions can affect the baby's disposition. In the Victorian era, women were instructed to avoid stressful thoughts and fill their minds with pleasant thoughts in order to have a happier baby. Some pieces of advice heard since then have been more specific. For example, pregnant women should not attend funerals or their babies may be sad and given to crying. Pregnant women should smile as much as possible in order to have babies that are smiley and happy.

There have, in fact, been many studies that demonstrate a link between mental states like depression and anxiety and its effects on offspring. It is often a difficult field to study because there are so many factors that can contribute to the outcome. If the baby of a woman who has depression in pregnancy has a bad temperament, is it the result of the woman's mood? Is it because she doesn't bond as well with the baby and provide it with a sense of protection? Is it a result of medications that she took while she was pregnant? Or is it a genetic tendency that predisposes some women to depression, and then gets passed on to the baby? Often it is hard to know what element of a woman's life has the most important influence on her baby's mental health.

The question may be partly answered by women who do not have a history of depression, but instead are exposed to extreme stress only during the pregnancy. When a woman experiences the loss of a partner, whether because he leaves her or dies, she is subject to major stress. Children born to women in these situations are more likely to have problems later in life such as depression, anxiety, or attention deficit disorder. Perhaps these changes can be attributed to the child growing up without two parents. However, a similar effect can be seen with women who experience the extreme stress of natural disasters during pregnancy. A study done in China evaluated children who were born shortly after a major earthquake hit the region.[14] These teenagers were found to have lower IQ scores on average than their peers who were born a year later. Similar effects were seen on children whose mothers had to endure a severe ice storm in Canada that resulted in many being displaced from their homes. These children had lower scores of intelligence and language abilities even at five years of age. These studies suggest that there may indeed be some adverse effect of subjecting pregnant women to extreme stress and anxiety. Perhaps the very large concentration of stress hormones like cortisol that are released in these situations can have lasting effects on the baby's brain development. However, these studies do not support the idea that pregnant women need to think happy thoughts all the time.

Though it may sound plausible that a mother can influence her baby's temperament by having a stressed state of mind, it seems far-fetched to think that thoughts can actually change the baby's appearance. Yet this belief is one that has been passed on throughout history, and is often heard even in this day and age. Historically, this idea has been termed "maternal impression," implying that a woman "impresses" or causes an imprint on the fetus through a strong thought. Sometimes the belief concerns a minor issue such as a birthmark. For example, a woman who craves strawberries while pregnant may have a child with a splotch on his arm in the shape of a strawberry. Sometimes, it is used to explain major birth defects. A woman whose baby is born with only one arm may think back and remember being frightened at some point during pregnancy by a man who also had only one arm. A famous story first told in ancient Greece but later appearing in medical texts two thousand years later told of an African queen whose light-skinned child was thought to be the result of the mother fixing her gaze on a white statue when she conceived. Perhaps this was an early way to explain why a baby could be an albino. Other stories relate situations where the baby looked nothing like the father because the mother was looking at a painting or statue during conception; these amusing tales sound like flimsy attempts at denying adultery, but they were earnestly believed by listeners two centuries ago.

Although one would think that these beliefs are just a remnant of the distant past, they still persist within recent generations. A 1978 survey of women receiving prenatal care at an urban clinic in Michigan found that 77 percent of the women interviewed thought it was possible to mark a baby through strong maternal emotions.[15] An Australian survey in 1971 found that 14 percent of women believed that maternal impression was possible.[16] Even in the twenty-first century, there are still some women who agree. A 2007 survey of women in Ohio found that 18 percent of women attending a clinic thought that pregnant women should avoid upsetting or violent images, and 5 percent felt that birth defects could be caused by seeing something ugly or frightening while pregnant.[17] It may be that these women are poorly educated, but it is disturbing to think that they may blame themselves for undesired pregnancy outcomes that are completely beyond anyone's control.

The origins of this belief date back at least to biblical times. In fact, the first known recorded example of maternal impression occurs in Genesis. When Jacob was working for his father-in-law Laban, Laban told Jacob that he could keep the cattle from his flock that were born with blemishes. Looking to keep as many cattle for himself as he could, Jacob set out speckled branches for the cows to see while they were mating. The implication is that these cows would have calves with mottled hides, since they were "impressed" by the vision of spotted branches. Since this story carried the weight of biblical authority, the idea that visual cues can affect a developing newborn was sustained in successive generations of Judeo-Christians.

Later writers continued to share stories of children affected in some way or another by their mothers' imaginations. The sixteenth-century surgeon Ambroise Pare wrote a whole book, *Monsters and Marvels*, about the various sorts of birth defects he had witnessed. He included a tale of a frog-faced boy whose mother conceived him after she "held a quicke frogge in her hand until it died."[18] A popular treatise on sex and pregnancy written at the end of the English Restoration period was called *Aristotle's Masterpiece*. It didn't actually have anything to do with the ancient Greek physician Aristotle, but since it bore his name, many were convinced that the ideas were from him. It, too, related stories of maternal impression, including a picture of a "maid all hairy" because her mother fixated on a painting of St. John the Baptist wearing a camel-hair shirt when she conceived.

The belief may have reached its peak of popularity in the early eighteenth century when a woman named Mary Toft achieved a degree of notoriety throughout England for claiming to have given birth to rabbits. According to Mary, she had a strong craving for rabbit meat while pregnant but was denied any to eat. She was so distraught and disappointed that she began to miscarry not one, but several rabbits. Her tale was so convincing that it attracted the attention of many noted physicians of the day, including the personal surgeon to King George I. He traveled to the small town where she lived to examine her and was convinced that she was telling the truth because he saw the rabbit parts emerge from her, and because he believed that such things were possible. Of course, she later admitted that she had inserted rabbit parts into her own vagina to carry out this ruse, but not until after several prominent physicians had weighed in on the matter.[19]

When the incident was demonstrated to be a fraud, the gullible physicians were mocked in popular cartoons and pamphlets. There were no tabloids in those days, but the attention given to this farce by the press gave Mary Toft the sort of infamy that would be created by tabloid covers today. By calling attention to such a ridiculous notion, that a woman could give birth to rabbits, the press also brought her doctors' medical judgment into question and caused widespread questioning of the concept of maternal impression.

Nevertheless, some physicians vigorously defended the idea, describing in great detail how maternal thought or fright may have an effect on fetal development. Daniel Turner, a member of London's College of Physicians, had published a tract titled "Spots and Marks of a Diverse Resemblance Imprest upon the Skin of the Foetus, by the Force of the Mother's Fancy." He engaged in a public debate with another member of the college, James Blondel, who published several works attacking this notion. Blondel logically argued that maternal impression could not possibly be true, giving many examples in his defense. He pointed out that vegetables often have blemishes, even though they have no conscience or imagination, and that seeing something frightening late in pregnancy could not possibly cause an entire arm or foot to magically disappear, as some people claimed was the cause for missing limbs.[20]

Many supporters of this idea continued to publish descriptions of maternal impression in medical books and journals through the eighteenth and nineteenth centuries. As principles of anatomy and pregnancy became more clearly understood, though, these authors became less and less convincing and more clear-thinking scientists tried to shut down this line of thinking. Critics pointed out that most of the cases of maternal impression were simply coincidental, based on a woman claiming that she had a thought or fright only after the child was born with a defect. Anyone, they argued, could come up with some memory over the course of nine months that could be linked to the birthmark in question. They also demonstrated that there was no connection of nerves between the mother and the fetus, so there would be no way for traumatic events in the mind of the mother to have any influence on the child growing within her. Even so, debate continued. One author in 1889 catalogued ninety cases of maternal impression reported in reputable medical journals between 1853 and 1886,[21] and an article discussing maternal impression appeared in the *Journal of the American Medical Association* in 1899.[22] By the end of the nineteenth century, authorities generally agreed that the idea of inducing birth defects in children through maternal mental anguish was hogwash.

Although it would seem that advances in science and medicine's embrace of more rational thought had put the notion to rest, a variation of the idea surfaced again in the 1960s. During this time, some observant epidemiologists noted an increased number of various birth defects in the children of women who had been subjected to great stress or "psychic trauma" in pregnancy. Examination of hospital records led some researchers to believe that defects such as extra fingers and toes, ear defects, cleft palate, and even Down syndrome (or "mongolism," as it was called at the time) were seen more often in children of mothers with emotional trauma. Could those imaginative physicians in the eighteenth century have been right? Could maternal emotions actually alter the child's appearance?

To test the theory, scientists experimented with mice. They exposed the pregnant mice to loud noises, or administered electric shocks over and over, until the mice displayed "nervous" behavior.[23] The mice who had been stressed delivered an unusually high number of babies with cleft palates in their litters. Scientists struggled with the idea of how one thing could cause the other. With no nerves communicating between the mother and the fetus, how could a stress or fright alter the baby's appearance? The theory was that these defects could be caused by high levels of cortisol, the so-called stress steroid, in the bloodstream of the affected animals. In fact, several studies demonstrated that cleft palates could be induced in mice just by injecting the mothers with high doses of cortisol.[24]

One may very well argue, however, that what goes on in the minds of rats is hardly the same as what human mothers experience. Causing a rodent to be flooded with cortisol by giving it shocks for days is a far cry from a surprising or traumatic experience of the sort that those early physicians thought would cause a defect in humans. Proving maternal impression in humans would involve experiments in which pregnant women would be repeatedly subjected to major stress and then looking for defective offspring. Of course it would be highly unethical to engineer such experiments in human subjects. No pregnant woman would subject herself to repetitive shocks or being repeatedly frightened to see if her baby would be born with a birth defect!

In situations where such experimentation is impossible, researchers often rely on population-based studies to look for a relationship between events and outcomes. By collecting information on large groups of people, epidemiologists can look for trends that would suggest a link between an event such as a stressful life event and an outcome such as a birth defect. Two large population-based studies that rely on large databases have done just that.

In Denmark, national registries are kept that contain personally identifiable information on every individual in the country who is born, dies, or gets hospitalized there. A study that examined hundreds of thousands of pregnancies over the course of over a decade examined the information linked between these registries in order to see which women were exposed to a "major stressor" during pregnancy.[25] The major stressors that were looked at were terrible life events, like having a child or spouse hospitalized during the pregnancy or experiencing the unexpected death of a child or spouse. The study showed that women with such exposure were about 50 percent more likely to have a child with a brain or head defect than unaffected women. The risk was highest in women who experienced a death of an older child while in their first trimester.

Another study was done looking at women in California who had delivered babies with birth defects.[26] The women were asked a series of questions about major life events such as death in the family, divorce, or episodes of violence, and their responses were compared with a control group of women who were similar demographically but had normal babies delivered over the same time period. The study demonstrated that the women whose babies had facial, brain, and heart anomalies were significantly more likely to have had major life stresses while pregnant. The study also showed that the risk became higher as the number of such stresses increased during pregnancy.

These and other similar studies suggest that major shocks and frights could actually have an effect on fetal development and lead to birth defects. These kinds of birth defects are rare, and the effect that was noted in these studies was small. Even if a particular defect was shown to be 50 percent more likely in women with a major stressful event in the first trimester, it would only account for less than one additional birth defect among one hundred babies born. So for the unfortunate woman who experiences the death of a loved one, she shouldn't also have to contend with the fear that she is likely to have an affected child.

Even with the evidence supporting this phenomenon, it does not exactly support the idea of maternal impression put forth in the previous centuries. The serious tragedies listed in the modern epidemiological studies were far worse than the sorts of minor events that eighteenth-century doctors advised against, like going without a food that was craved or seeing an injured man on the street. So those historical physicians who supported maternal impression were not particularly observant, and these stressful life events were not what they had in mind. Still, those old wives who tell women not to attend funerals while they are pregnant may not be entirely wrong.

The bottom line is that bad things like miscarriages and birth defects can and do happen under the best of circumstances, and most of the time they are beyond anyone's control. In general, the best advice for women who want a healthy baby is to stay healthy, exercise, and try to minimize the stress in their lives as much as possible.

7

LENGTH OF PREGNANCY

One of the first questions that women ask after finding out they are pregnant is "When is the baby due?" Estimating the expected arrival time is important for both social and medical reasons. Women need to know when the baby will arrive so they can plan when to take time off, when to make arrangements for child care, and when to have family come to provide assistance. They may want the answer to start a mental countdown toward the joyous day of childbirth, or they may start counting the days until the discomforts and nuisances of pregnancy will end. Health care experts need to know the expected due date so that they can gauge how well the baby is growing, anticipate any changes that might indicate premature labor, and monitor the pregnancy to ensure it doesn't go on too long and put the baby at risk. For some women, the issue of gestational age has serious implications for paternity; if the baby is due nine months after her husband was away on business for a month, a woman may have some explaining to do! Many of the myths and old wives' tales surrounding due dates do not have much to do with advice or recommendations. Nevertheless, there are several ideas and misconceptions that women share about due dates that fall under the folklore theme.

One common misconception is that a due date is a hard and fast line to cross. Women who are given a date when the baby is "due" might compare it to the due date on a library book. That is, they assume that the baby had better come by that time, and if she doesn't, then the baby is overdue and will need to be evicted. In reality, the due date is only an estimation of when the baby is expected, and a two-week window on either side of that date is considered fair game for guessing when labor will actually start. Health care providers refer to the date as an "estimated date of delivery," or the more antiquated term "estimated date of confinement," to emphasize that it is really just a guess and not a firm commitment.

Knowing when to expect the baby to come has not always been an easy guess. The date that labor begins involves various factors including the time of conception, the genetic predisposition of the baby, and mechanical factors that influence the forces on the uterus and the cervix. Nowadays, doctors rely on sonograms done early in pregnancy to pinpoint exactly how far along the pregnancy is and when the woman is likely to have conceived. Furthermore, health professionals have a good understanding of when ovulation occurs relative to a woman's menstrual cycle and can use this information to get a handle on when conception occurred.

Thousands of years ago, the picture was not so clear. Ancient physicians recognized that typical pregnancies lasted about nine months, but they gave considerable leeway as to the minimum and maximum length. The discrepancies in reporting how long it took from the previous menstrual period until delivery were accounted for by stating that different babies could take different amounts of time to develop. Some babies, it was felt, were ready after seven months; others took ten months to develop fully. These parameters were sufficient to explain most cases where either paternity or legitimacy was in question. If the couple had their baby only seven months after the marriage took place, then that must be one of those quickly developing babies!

Babies that were born after only eight months, however, were a special case.[1] Many ancient sources considered these infants to be nonviable and sure to die at birth or shortly after. Ancient Greek writers including Hippocrates, Herodotus, and Galen agreed that while a child born after only seven months of pregnancy could survive, an eight-month baby never did. The reasons for this belief were mostly numerological, since the number 7 was seen as having lucky and magical properties, while 8 did not. The Hippocratic doctrine on the subject explains that fetuses grow in strength in the seventh month, but both the fetus and mother suffer illness or pain in the eighth month and take another month to recover fully. This treatise maintains that it is also dangerous for the mother's health to deliver in the eighth month. Perhaps this belief was useful in explaining situations where either infants or mothers died after a complicated early delivery, since it helped to shift blame away from the birth attendant.

Regardless of the reason for its origin, this belief has been strangely persistent.[2] The idea that eight-month babies do not survive is mentioned in medieval medical texts and also by Renaissance writers in France and Great Britain. Beyond that, the idea has not been given serious consideration by the medical establishment. It is still mentioned even in this century, though, by mothers who face the prospect of having their babies prematurely. Mothers from various backgrounds have asked their obstetricians to induce labor in the face of an early pregnancy complication so that the baby could be born in the seventh month rather than the eighth one. For example, a woman with severely high blood pressure at 29 weeks asked to have her baby delivered soon so that it would not risk delivery in the eighth month. Of course, there is no medical reason to substantiate such a request. It is well known that babies are more likely to survive with the fewest possible complications the closer they are born to the due date. This seems to be an example of an old wives' tale that has filtered down from ancient medicine despite a lack of any evidence to support it.

Another such belief has to do with how quickly babies are formed. Several comments on Internet websites mention how boys are thought to form earlier than girls. Such postings mention how they can predict the gender of the fetus based on early ultrasounds in the first trimester. The writers report that they have been told that boys take on distinct features earlier than girls do, so if there are clearly visible hands and feet at this stage, the fetus must be male.

This notion also dates back to the ancient Greeks. Aristotle wrote that the male embryo was completely formed by 40 days of gestation, and this is when the soul entered the child. Girls, he said, took longer to develop and remained undifferentiated and unformed until 90 days of gestation.[3] The idea persisted with some minor changes in Judaic tradition as well. Rabbi Ishmael wrote in the Mishnah, a collection of Jewish oral traditions from the early centuries of the Christian era, that a male fetus is fully formed after 41 days, but a female fetus is not finished until day 81.[4] The exact number of days may be in question, but it seems that the prevailing sentiment was that girls were slower and took longer to develop.

Today, we know that fetal development occurs at the same rate in both genders and identifying the gender on ultrasound cannot be done reliably until the second trimester. There is still some concern voiced by expectant parents that girls do take longer to "get ready." These parents claim that if a woman is expecting a daughter, her labor is likely to start later. Whether due to some remnant of these ancient beliefs, or just due to gender stereotyping, the impression remains that girls keep parents waiting longer than boys.

For the most part, this idea is unfounded. Among pregnancies where mothers reach their due dates, labor begins at the same time whether the mother is carrying a boy or a girl.[5] In fact, there is some evidence that in those women who go considerably past the due date, it may be boys who keep the parents waiting. One study showed that among women who went all the way to 43 weeks (which admittedly does not happen very often), there were three male babies for every two females born.[6] So at least in some circumstances, it may take boys a little longer to get ready after all.

At the other end of the late pregnancy spectrum, there is a very different effect of gender. Among babies that are born prematurely, before 37 weeks of gestation, boys outnumber the girls. A Swedish study of premature births showed that among babies delivered before 32 weeks, 55 percent were male and 45 percent were female.[7] The difference was even more profound for the most premature babies. The reasons for this are not well understood. It may have something to do with a gender difference in placental function, or how boy fetuses react to stressors like infection or inflammation differently from girls. In either case, the likelihood that a boy baby will deliver prematurely is significantly greater.

However, when a girl is born prematurely, she tends to do better than her male counterpart delivered at exactly the same age. Female infants that are born prematurely are less likely to have lung complications or difficulty breathing and have overall higher survival rates.[8] This survival advantage is in part due to the fact that baby girls' lungs develop faster in the womb and are more likely to produce the chemicals that enable them to breathe air. So in this respect, the ancients had it wrong.

It seems that girls actually do develop and mature a little faster than boys.

Despite subtle differences in gender, it is still commonly accepted that it takes nine months for the fetus to completely mature. In anticipating when to expect the baby to emerge, women are eager to learn of an exact due date. As mentioned earlier, this date may be assigned by a health care practitioner based on data from the woman's menstrual history or a sonogram. Prior to seeing a provider, women may try to calculate the date on their own. A common piece of advice that is shared among women is to calculate the due date by subtracting three months from the start of the last menstrual period and adding seven days. For example, if a woman began her last period on April 9, her due date would be January 16.

This piece of advice is not an old wives' tale but is based on a medical principle known as "Naegele's rule."[9] Franz Carl Naegele was a nineteenth-century German professor of obstetrics who published his assessment in 1812. He based his rule on a much older set of observations. He referenced the work of a Dutch physician, Hermann Boerhaave, who worked out the calculation of pregnancy length in the early eighteenth century. He speculated that a pregnancy should last ten lunar months, or 280 days, based on observations and a reckoning of the biblical account of Mary's pregnancy. Since this was the length of time from the Feast of the Annunciation in March until Christmas Day in December, this should be the standard length of human gestation. The observation, as it turned out, was pretty close to the truth and has widely been accepted as the basis for calculating due dates right up to the present day.

To be exact, though, Naegele and his colleagues were just slightly off. Large population-based studies, such as an examination of the Swedish birth registry involving 427,582 pregnancies,[10] show that human pregnancies with one fetus are on average just a tiny bit longer. This study showed an average length of 281 days, but a modal duration of 283 days. The mode (or most common single number of days on record) was felt to be the most accurate for a typical pregnancy, as it tends to reduce the influence of abnormal pregnancies at the far ends of the distribution. So both the old wives and their doctors may want to consider adding a couple of days to the calculated due date to avoid unnecessary worry when the baby arrives a few days "overdue."

A final rumor that many women share about when to expect their little ones has to do with birth order. A common piece of folklore that is circulated among expectant women is that the first baby tends to be late, while subsequent deliveries will come earlier. This observation is not based on any ancient medical texts. It most likely derives from the greater anxiety and lack of experience that first-time mothers may feel as the due date approaches. In other words, when you are waiting for your first baby, it may seem like it is taking forever; when you are busy caring for other children and not as fearful of what labor will be like, you may not notice how slowly the days creep by.

The evidence for this prediction is mixed. Websites in support of the assertion point to a study that analyzed data from over nine thousand births at a single hospital in Boston.[11] The authors suggested that women who had given birth before had shorter pregnancies on average than first-time mothers. However, the data came from births between 1977 and 1980, before most women had sonograms to confirm when they actually got pregnant. More recent assessments have been circulated on the Internet. One unpublished study analyzed data from a national database with information on over thirty thousand pregnancies that resulted in a live birth.[12] The author found a very slight difference, with first babies arriving on average at 38.61 weeks and other babies at 38.52 weeks. Although this represents less than a day's difference, it was statistically significant. The trouble with this assessment is that it included premature births, as well as inductions, which are often scheduled prior to the due date for women who have given birth before.

Another Internet study examined the question in 11,900 women who responded to a survey about pregnancy length.[13] This study excluded women who labored before 35 weeks of pregnancy and also excluded induced births. There was no difference in the pregnancy length of first births and subsequent births: both were 278 days. Furthermore, the analysis included a look at the experience of individual mothers. That is, for each woman, the author plotted when her first delivery occurred relative to her second. She found that the average baby number two came 0.42 days later than its older sibling. It seems safe to say that an average pregnant woman need not fear that she will be kept waiting longer just because it is her first time at bat.

The bottom line for mothers waiting for their babies to arrive is that it takes as long as it takes. Barring a situation where there is a medical reason to anticipate an early delivery, babies come sometime around the nine-month mark, and there is considerable variation that is difficult to anticipate. In any case, the old wives and their ancient sources don't have much to add to this simple philosophy.

8

INDUCING LABOR

Finally, after months of waiting and hoping, the due date approaches! Along with the growing anticipation of finally getting to welcome the long-awaited baby come other growing features. Ankles swell, the back aches, and bladder capacity dwindles. It becomes difficult to put on shoes or even rise from a chair. It is no wonder that many women wish there were a way to put an end to all the miserable aches and pains by moving up the delivery date. Even though gestation has a finite "term limit," the growing frustration with waiting for labor to start encourages many women to try to take the matter into their own hands.

Women looking for help in how to bring on labor will find plenty of options listed on pregnancy websites and Internet chat rooms. The list of recommendations that women share on this subject is long, and it seems that everyone has an anecdote about what she was doing before her baby came that must have been the trick that brought on the contractions. Based on the number of websites geared toward sharing these recommendations, there is a large audience of women eager to find out how to make their pregnancy a little bit shorter. Indeed, a survey of women who had just given birth in one hospital demonstrated that a majority did something to try to bring on labor themselves.[1] Women who were hospitalized after delivery were asked if they had participated in any one of a dozen activities for the sole purpose of bringing on labor, and 102 out of 201 women had done so in the prior week. The most common techniques that they volunteered were extra walking and having sex, and the most common source for these recom-

mendations was friends and family. Regardless of the source of information or the type of activity that was mentioned, the plan to bring on
labor a little early was expressed by women of all different backgrounds,
educational levels, and ages.

Advice on getting labor to start is nothing new, and these pieces of
folklore reflect a long history of puzzling over how to get the process
started. Various cultures and groups through history have had ideas
about what factors will hasten delivery. A common theme, particularly
among primitive peoples, is the idea that the baby itself is the one to
initiate delivery.[2] If the baby is happy growing in the mother's womb, it
is likely to stay put. So by making the uterine environment a place
where the baby would be less comfortable, the mother may be able to
coax the baby to come out.

One way to do so would be to starve the baby out. Among certain
Native American tribes it was common for a woman to fast during the
week prior to her anticipated delivery so that the baby would be hungry
and eager to emerge to take the mother's milk.[3] The Paiutes believed
this had a dual purpose because it would also reduce the amount of fat
tissue around the genital organs to give the baby a wider berth. The
hungry fetus would also cause the uterus to start to contract so that the
labor would get started.

Nowadays, we scoff at the idea that a baby can "decide" to come out
just because it is hungry. Nevertheless, it has been observed that wom-
en who do not eat regularly are at risk of going into labor early. A survey
of women's dietary habits in North Carolina demonstrated that women
who fell short of the recommended three-meals-a-day diet during their
second trimester were 30 percent more likely to deliver prematurely.[4]
The authors theorized that these women may have been under more
stress, which could have brought on early delivery.

Whether starvation could actually initiate labor is a hard theory to
test. Asking women not to eat is ethically questionable and probably not
good for the developing fetus. An interesting paper that might lend
some support to the theory, however, was written in Israel.[5] The authors reported on what they called the "Yom Kippur effect." In the
Jewish religion, men and women traditionally go without food or drink
for a 24-hour period on Yom Kippur, the holiest day of the Jewish
calendar. The authors noted that in the 24-hour period following Yom
Kippur, there was a statistically significant increase in the number of

babies born in Jerusalem. Even if starvation does contribute to the onset of labor, it is not a healthy or comfortable practice for full-term women.

How else might women have made the baby want to come out? Some other practices involved more physical discomfort to make the baby want to leave the womb to avoid pain. Sometimes it was just by threat of physical pain. There are accounts of labor assistants yelling at the fetus and threatening it if it would not emerge. Another Native American practice was for a pregnant woman to sit alone on the prairie while a horseman galloped toward her with the appearance of imminently trampling her. Of course, he would veer aside at the last minute, but the fear of imminent harm would supposedly start labor.

Other techniques sound more painful. A pregnant woman whose fetus was viewed as overstaying its welcome might be bounced in a blanket, suspended upside down and shaken, or have a sash tied tightly around the upper abdomen to force the baby out.[6] No woman today would subject herself to such harsh treatment, which sounds far worse than the discomfort of being pregnant for a few more days. But there are echoes of these ideas in modern practice. Thirty percent of women in a recent survey believed that strenuous exercise or exertion could hasten labor, and a few recommended activities such as dancing or going for a ride over a bumpy road to shake the baby out of its comfy home.[7] A seventeenth-century obstetrics text noted that many midwives of the day advised women who were due to ride in coaches or on trotting horses in order to loosen the bonds that held the baby in place, though the author recognized that such recommendations were "dangerous advice."[8]

In general, shaking and pregnancy don't mix well. There is a reason why signs at amusement parks forbid pregnant women from going on thrill rides. Rapid changes in acceleration or force on the pregnant uterus can cause the placenta to separate from the uterine wall, leading to bleeding or even fetal death. So bumpy roads and jumping up and down are probably not good ideas. For more restrained forms of exercise and movement, the evidence is more controversial.

Studies looking at women who exercise in pregnancy show mixed results. One study looked at women who were fit and exercised regularly prior to pregnancy.[9] The women who gave up exercise early in pregnancy tended to deliver on average six days later than the ones who continued to exercise throughout their pregnancies. On the other hand, a study of 1,647 women in North Carolina demonstrated that those who engaged regularly in vigorous recreational activity delivered later than their counterparts who were inactive.[10] In either case, the research examined women who were exercising regularly and remaining physically fit, so the findings would not apply to the inactive woman who decides that she will spend an hour on the treadmill just to get labor started. There may indeed be benefits of exercise during pregnancy, but avoiding a longer pregnancy is not one of them.

A milder form of exercise that is perhaps the most frequently mentioned technique for starting labor is walking. It is very common to hear from the woman who is past her due date, "I don't understand why I haven't gone into labor yet. I've been walking and walking all week!" In the survey mentioned earlier, 87 of the 102 women who confessed to doing something just to bring on labor before birth said they had tried walking.[11] In another survey asking women immediately postpartum what had started their labor, 32 percent thought that going for a walk was the trick that got the baby to come out.[12]

Although walking is strongly believed to be a trigger for labor by the lay public, medical evidence is scant. There is no study comparing when labor starts for women who walk a lot or a little. The only information that may be relevant is what is known about walking once labor has already started. In women who are given the option of walking during the early part of labor or resting in bed, there is no particular benefit for the walkers in terms of faster labor.[13] However, some small studies have suggested a benefit of walking for women who are making slow progress in the early part of labor. However, none of these studies suggest that walking will start the labor process. If a woman feels like walking as she gets close to her due date, she should be allowed to do so as a healthy and gentle form of exercise. But she should not expect that it will make the baby come any sooner.

If the baby can't be shaken loose by exercise or activity, another thought that impatient mothers have had is to try to start labor by stimulating the intestinal tract. Various substances have been suggested that might bring on labor through a laxative effect. The thought process goes something like this: forcing one thing out through the bottom is likely to have an effect on forcing other things out. So if the rectum can be stimulated to eject its contents, perhaps the uterus will, too.

It's not clear whether this line of thinking has much of a history. It may be an example of "imitative magic," the sort of folklore where one activity is thought to cause another because of a perceived similarity. It may also be an example of practice based on observation. It was a common practice in seventeenth- and eighteenth-century medicine to administer purgatives for a host of medical disorders. An obstetrician of the early nineteenth century noted that the use of purgatives in pregnancy can be dangerous because it may stimulate abortion in early pregnancy or premature labor, due to "the strong consent between the uterus and rectum."[14] In fact, he noted, labor will often start with an episode of diarrhea, though he would not recommend the use of laxatives as a means of causing labor.

To this day, however, there are many who do. The most commonly recommended and studied form of laxative is castor oil. It is unclear when castor oil was first used as an agent to induce labor. The ancient Egyptians recognized it as a laxative, but there is nothing written in their texts to suggest it was used for the purpose of inducing labor. Nevertheless, it was in common usage by the medical community throughout the early part of the twentieth century and is mentioned in medical textbooks of obstetrics.[15] It fell out of favor midcentury, probably because of the success and availability of oxytocin, which is the pituitary hormone primarily used in hospitals today for labor induction. That oxytocin has enjoyed a successful run since then does not make those earlier successes with castor oil any less real. However, it was not until recently that the effects of castor oil were examined with any reliable research.

There have been two randomized, controlled trials of castor oil for labor induction. In other words, these studies assigned women who were waiting to go into labor to either use a measured amount of castor oil, or to have no treatment, and then see how long it would take for labor to start. In one of these studies,[16] the women had all passed their due dates and were otherwise healthy. Fifty-eight percent of women who used castor oil went into labor within 24 hours, compared to only 4 percent who used nothing. In the other study,[17] women who had ruptured their membranes at full term but had not started labor were included. In that study again, significantly more women went into labor after taking castor oil, though the effect was not quite as dramatic. These studies suggest that this is a folk remedy that does, in fact, work.

Many practitioners continue to recommend the use of castor oil, although references are much more common in journals read by midwives than in medical journals. Part of the reluctance on the part of physicians to embrace this method stems from the fact that unregulated administration of castor oil may have some bad effects.[18] Just as this remedy causes diarrhea in the mother, there is some concern that it can cross the placenta and make the fetus have a bowel movement, too. There have been reports that babies of mothers who take castor oil may be more likely to have bowel contents (called meconium) in the amniotic fluid that the baby might inhale during birth. There was also a report of a mother sustaining brain damage from a severe pregnancy complication known as amniotic fluid embolism after she took castor oil. The cause of this event was not proven, but the link in time between the two events certainly gives cause for caution.

Not only might the use of such a laxative be dangerous, but the idea of subjecting a woman to the discomforts of diarrhea on top of the discomforts of nine months of pregnancy is unappealing. Not to mention that the taste of castor oil is very unpleasant. Some more appealing substances have more recently been suggested as possible induction agents—particularly if one likes spicy food, since that is now most commonly recommended to promote labor.

The Internet is rife with suggestions by various culinary establishments that their spicy dish is the one that will make pregnant women deliver. Spicy Chinese dishes, Indian food, and eggplant parmigiana are all entrees that have been touted as having some effect in causing contractions. The idea is not so much to cause diarrhea as it is to promote intestinal peristalsis. That is, spicy food may be somewhat irritating to the gut and get it to move and squeeze its contents more forcefully. Of course, none of these restaurants have done any studies to prove that their offerings actually trigger labor, but the baby pictures that they post on the walls provide the "proof" that their dishes work.

Interestingly, there was a study that provides some evidence for the link between spicy food and labor. In a group of women admitted to the hospital because of preterm labor (before the baby is ready for arrival), a survey was given to see what factors they had been exposed to in the day just before admission.[19] The factor with the strongest association was eating something spicy within 24 hours before labor began. Skipping a meal was also noted to increase the odds of going into labor.

Since these women were well ahead of their due dates, the findings may not apply to women at term who are trying to start labor. Of course, a woman who is past her due date and hoping to deliver soon might go into labor regardless of how many jalapenos she adds to her plate. Furthermore, there is no evidence that women in countries like India or Thailand, where food tends to be spicier, have pregnancies that are any shorter than women in cultures that dine on blander foods. Still, if a woman has a strong stomach and a taste for spicy cuisine, it wouldn't hurt to try adding some pepper to her dinner.

Another addition to the menu that might be a little easier to take is pineapple. Recommending pineapple for getting labor under way is a relatively new piece of folklore that has been circulated more frequently in the past few years. There is no mention of it in Western historical writings, which is hardly surprising given that pineapples are native to tropical climates and would not have been easily available to most women in the Western world. In India and Bangladesh, however, it has been used as part of traditional medicine for women who want to miscarry. The issue that makes this recommendation somewhat plausible is that pineapples contain a compound called bromelain that may stimulate muscular contractions in a laboratory.[20] The amount is small, though, and in order to ingest enough bromelain to have a possible effect on her uterus, a woman would have to eat seven to eight whole pineapples. Though some women may find pineapples to be a tasty solution, this serving size would likely result only in a huge amount of sugar intake and maybe diarrhea (which could have an effect for other reasons previously mentioned).

Another recommendation that is very commonly heard by pregnant women eager to get labor started involves what happens after dinner is over. "Have some spicy Chinese food, and then have sex" is advice that women claim to have heard from physicians and girlfriends alike. Having sexual intercourse to induce labor is a popular idea, with 74 percent of pregnant women in one survey having heard this advice.[21] Among postpartum women who were asked what they had done the previous week to get labor started, 23 percent reported having sex for this purpose.[22] Perhaps this notion is particularly popular because sex is a much more appealing option than laxatives, exercise, or starvation. Or could it be popular because it actually works?

The idea is popular not just among the "civilized" world of pregnancy chat rooms. Surveys in other cultures demonstrate a widespread view that coitus may facilitate labor by mechanical means. The penis, according to these proponents, acts as a dilator that widens the vaginal opening (and thus the "birth canal"), allowing for an easier labor. Surveys of women in such disparate areas as Nigeria,[23] Pakistan, [24] and Jamaica [25] have demonstrated that this is a common belief in these communities. A dilator the size of a penis is not going to have much of an effect on creating room for something the size of a baby, but this widespread concept is more symbolic than practical and still offers an excuse to engage in some intimacy before the baby crashes the party.

Antiquarian medical books are generally mute on this subject, since doctors of old were not likely to recommend induction of labor and usually only brought up sex during pregnancy when discouraging it. It may be that women noticed an increase in contractions following orgasm, which has been shown to involve contractions of both the uterus and pelvic floor in medical studies. They or their doctors may have drawn the conclusion that if contractions occur with sex, then labor may result.

Whatever the origin, the idea has drawn much attention from both the medical and lay communities due to its plausibility. It seems plausible not only because the contractions that may be noticed after orgasm mimic the uterine contractions that contribute to labor. There is also a theoretical relationship between starting labor and the components of semen that are introduced during ejaculation. Seminal fluid is known to contain compounds known as prostaglandins of the same type as those used by physicians to induce labor. These chemicals serve to "ripen" the cervix, or render it softer and easier to dilate in the setting of contractions. The idea that there is a natural (and fun!) way to deposit those compounds right at the cervix where they could help the labor process may justify the attempts of women trying to get labor started by having sex.

As scientific as it sounds, though, there is little evidence to show that it actually works. In one study, cervical exams of women who did and did not engage in sexual intercourse were compared from week to week at the very end of their pregnancies.[26] Not only did the cervix not ripen or change more in the sexually active women, but those women who had had sex delivered on average three days later than the women who did not. Of course, there are many factors that go into the decision to have sex, and the women who did not have sex may have delivered earlier because they were also the ones who were crampier, more uncomfortable, and just getting ready to go into labor anyway. Two more studies tried to eliminate this bias by randomizing the participants who were having sex.[27] In other words, as much as such a thing can be controlled, the participants were either told randomly to have sex in order to hasten the labor process, or left to their own devices. These studies, too, failed to show any difference in the onset of labor between the two groups.

Another activity related to sexual intercourse may contribute to some of the conversations about sex bringing on labor. A woman's breasts may be stimulated either as part of foreplay or during a sexual encounter. Stimulation of the nipples is known to release the hormone oxytocin from the pituitary gland. This hormone helps in milk letdown once a woman is nursing and helps the uterus to contract back to its normal size following delivery. It is also the hormone that is most frequently used to induce labor. So it makes perfect sense that stimulating the nipples should have a legitimate effect in triggering labor contractions.

Several studies have supported this theory. When comparing women who stimulated the nipples during a medical induction of labor with those who relied on medicine alone, researchers have demonstrated a positive effect of nipple stimulation on the success of induction and the length of labor. A summary of the research on this subject concluded that nipple stimulation results in more women going into labor within 72 hours than women who do nothing.[28] This would seem to be an effective technique in getting labor to start a little sooner than nature intended. However, this method may work a little too well. The strength of contractions that result from nipple stimulation may be quite powerful, and it is possible for the uterus to contract too much. This kind of excessive contraction, known as uterine hyperstimulation, can cause a decrease in blood flow to the baby and possibly even fetal injury. So nipple stimulation should not be recommended unless the effect of the intervention can be properly monitored.

Since asking women about recent sexual activity usually does not specify whether massage or stroking of breasts was involved, it is hard to know how much of the rumors about sex and induction are due to vaginal sex and how much are due to stimulation in general. Still the majority of research does not support any utility of sexual intercourse in promoting labor. There are plenty of other good reasons to have sex, though, and it may be a fine way to pass the time until the baby arrives.

Many other potential therapies have been talked about in one forum or another as nonmedical ways that a woman can bring on labor.[29] Herbal teas, reflexology, aromatherapy, flower remedies, and hypnosis are all techniques that women may hear about as methods to take matters into their own hands when pregnancy seems to be going on too long. None of them have been proven effective. In most cases, there is very little that women can do to change the preordained time for their children to be born. It would seem that labor is a phenomenon whose onset is still a mystery, and a woman has little control over when it occurs.

This sense of mystery and lack of control may be the reason that women sometimes thought natural phenomena played a role in the labor process. In looking to the heavens and wondering when labor will start, some women have thought they found an answer in the moon shining back. In fact, people have drawn a relationship between the moon and birth since ancient times.[30] In Greek, Celtic, and Babylonian mythology, the goddesses associated with the moon were also given a role of watching over childbirth. It's only a coincidence that it takes twenty-nine days for the moon to go through a cycle of its phases, which is about the same amount of time between a woman's menstrual periods. Yet in many cultures, this coincidence has led to the belief that the moon controls the uterus, and changes in the moon can affect a woman's ability to reproduce.

Modern women are not likely to be worshiping moon goddesses or even timing their fertile moments by watching the moon. But there is a persistent myth that labor may be tied to the full moon. Many women are told that they are more likely to go into labor when the moon is full. This is a particularly popular saying among labor floor nurses, who commonly predict that their shift will be busy if it falls on the night of a full moon. A survey of nurses on one labor unit noted that 68 percent believed that labor is more likely to start during a full moon.[31]

With that sort of authoritative support, one might think that such an effect is well documented. In fact, the link between phases of the moon and the onset of labor has been disproved over and over. There is nearly a century of research on labor floor records and how they relate to the moon's changes. Even though there have been comprehensive reviews showing no association, more papers keep popping up in the medical literature.[32] Could it be that the influence is only there at night? Or that it only would be noticed in remote areas free from the artificial lights of industrialized society? No and no, as subsequent research has shown. Yet the regularity with which such research is done demonstrates that there are scientists out there who will not let go of the question. The idea that the moon influences the course of our lives is so embedded in the human psyche that many doctors and patients alike continue to believe that a full moon creates a busy labor floor despite overwhelming evidence to the contrary.

Another natural phenomenon that many people link to labor is stormy weather. "There's a big storm brewing" is a prediction that labor floor nurses do not like to hear. For one thing, it implies that they may have a difficult time getting to work. What they fear more is that a bad storm portends a heavier than usual workload on the labor floor. Why this belief is popular is hard to say. Unlike the long history of folklore surrounding the moon, there is no historical equivalent when it comes to weather. Authors who write about this link mostly claim that they explore the topic because of anecdotal evidence, where someone noticed a particularly busy day when a cloudburst occurred. Some have tried to justify the relationship by relating labor to atmospheric pressure. They compare the amniotic sac that holds the baby within to a balloon, and theorize what may happen when pressure changes on the outside of that balloon. Since balloons expand when the atmospheric pressure around them drops, it might make sense that the amniotic sac may be more likely to expand when the barometric pressure falls. Like a balloon popping when it gets too big, the amniotic sac would then rupture, which is what women refer to as "breaking water." Since labor almost always follows soon after membrane rupture at the end of pregnancy, this change in the weather could be an indirect trigger of labor pains.

Despite the plausibility of this argument, the evidence is not very supportive. Two very large studies looked at population data and meteorological data in Massachusetts[33] and Arizona,[34] two areas with very different weather. Both agreed, though, that there was no significant difference in the number of women who went into labor following drops in atmospheric pressure. Studies that have looked only at rupture of membranes, however, have been more supportive. A group of researchers in Iowa compared the birth records of women who lived in a single 100-mile radius.[35] They found that women in this area who had broken their water before labor started were more likely to have done so within three hours after a major drop in the atmospheric pressure. Another study in Athens, Greece, also suggested a statistically significant relationship between membrane rupture and a falling barometer, but accounting for only a slight change in the number of hospital admissions.[36] There may be a grain of truth to this idea, but chasing storms would be an unreliable way for a woman interested in moving up her delivery date to initiate labor.

So what is an uncomfortable and impatient pregnant woman at the end of nine months to do? There are few recommendations that may actually help to get labor started. Castor oil and nipple stimulation seem to have the most evidence for being effective, but there is some risk to using them as well. Walking and sex may be done for enjoyment but probably will not move up the due date. As for spicy food, there is not much evidence that it will help, but it probably doesn't hurt (if you don't count a burning tongue as painful).

Of course, there are a variety of drugs and tools to initiate labor when the need arises. Physicians and midwives may use these safe and reliable treatments when there is a medical reason for delivering the baby, before either the mother or the infant suffers from prolonging a potentially dangerous situation. However, these medical situations demand induction when there is a clear opinion that the baby will do better outside of the womb than inside. That is not the case when labor induction is considered because the mother is sick of dealing with swollen ankles, or just tired of being tired. In general, the baby decides when it is the right time to emerge, and labor doesn't start until the baby is ready and fully mature. Even if the occasional folk remedy has been shown to make labor start sooner, the healthiest and safest course for most women is to let the baby come in its own sweet time.

9

EASING LABOR

Most women look forward to their due dates with keen anticipation. They know that when they finally give birth, there will be an end to months of discomfort, and they will have a beautiful baby to love and enjoy. As for the actual birth process, though, they may not be so keen. When women speak of the labor experience, descriptions of pain are usually given top billing. Women often hear horror stories about the length and intensity of pain, and even about complications that can cause injury to the laboring woman or her baby. With all the planning that goes on for how and when the baby will come, most women can only hope and pray for a labor that will be smooth and relatively quick. It is no wonder, then, that many pieces of folklore have been passed along about how to make the labor process an easier one.

Folklore dealing with labor is as old as recorded history. Some of the earliest examples of human writing are from ancient Mesopotamia. Cuneiform tablets from this civilization over four thousand years ago contain instructions on how women can overcome difficulty in childbirth.[1] The Ebers papyrus from ancient Egypt, written about 1550 BCE, also suggests a number of remedies for making childbirth go smoothly. In ancient times, childbirth was seen as being inherently dangerous and led to tragic circumstances for either the mother or infant (or both) in a small but greatly feared percentage of cases. Even today, childbirth remains a dangerous and often feared event for women in cultures and geographical regions with no access to medical care or informed supervision. Many of the folkloric themes that began many years ago are still echoed in recommendations heard today.

Some of the more primitive recommendations that exist on this subject are shaped by the symbolism that is tied to childbirth. In essence, childbirth involves fitting a rather large object through a relatively narrow opening. The birth canal is viewed as a passageway, and an obstructed birth and long labor could be a consequence of anything that would make that passage narrower or closed. Consequently, many of the recommendations involve simply keeping things open. Examples in cultures from around the world emphasize the importance of opening or unlocking.[2] No one should stand in the doorway where a pregnant woman is giving birth. Clothing that is fastened with knots should be untied. Hair that is braided should be undone and worn loose. Doors, closets, and drawers are to be left wide open. Some have even recommended that horses should be set loose from the stable and fowl allowed to roam free when labor is progressing slowly. One can only imagine the outrageous scene that might have greeted some poor laboring woman with barnyard animals running through all those open doors!

Other pieces of advice have been symbolic in a similar vein. A Finnish custom instructs a wife to crawl between the legs of her drunken husband on the eve of her wedding day in order to ensure that her births will be easy. Other superstitions rely on the idea of pain as something that can be literally cut. The *Farmers' Almanac* recommends placing a sharp knife under the bed of a laboring woman to cut the pain,[3] and some tales specify that it should be an axe laid down with the sharp blade pointing up toward the woman resting above.

These symbolic gestures are an example of "magical thinking," in which the participant hopes that she will cause a change in something by manipulating a proxy for that thing. This kind of advice is usually restricted to cultures and places where the birth process is poorly understood.[4] Perhaps some well-meaning birth attendants have engaged in these activities as harmless ways to bide their time and try to be helpful. It is probably not because any of these methods have been observed to really change the birth process. No modern-day medical practitioner would take seriously the instructions to untie clothing, nor would she perform an experiment to see if such a precaution is useful.

Yet the idea of avoiding being bound finds some parallel in the advice that is sometimes heard on labor floors today. Women who labor in hospital settings are often confined to a hospital bed, with their abdomen encircled by bands with monitors attached that track the fetal heartbeat pattern. Using these monitors, obstetricians are able to continuously watch how the fetus responds to contractions and to the medications used in labor. These cords and monitors help to make sure that the baby remains healthy through the stresses of labor. However, many contemporary "old wives" object to this practice, arguing that forcing a woman to be "tied down" to the bed and unable to move about freely could slow down the labor or worsen the pain.

While tying and untying hair braids does not seem like a suitable subject of a medical experiment, this kind of binding makes more sense for experimentation. Several research studies have been done to look at whether there is an advantage to allowing women to walk or move freely during her labor. A review of studies that examined unrestricted movement in the first stage of labor (that is, before women were ready to push) found that women who were allowed to walk and remain upright had shorter labors and lower rates of Cesarean than women who were kept lying down.[5] This review also suggested that women are less likely to get an epidural for pain if they are able to continue walking. Perhaps it is the epidural for these women and not the forced bed rest that affected the length of labor. In a separate study that looked only at women who had an epidural in the first stage of labor, there was no difference in any birth outcome or satisfaction with pain relief between those who were able to walk and those who did not.[6] Sometimes a laboring woman is told to stay on the monitor for other reasons. This decision, which affects how restricted a woman's movement might be, could be based on factors that determine how risky it would be for her to get off the monitor. For example, in cases where the labor is being induced due to problems in the baby, or the pregnancy is complicated by the mother's medical condition, continuous monitoring might be necessary to make sure the baby remains healthy through labor. But the evidence suggests that in uncomplicated low-risk labors, women should be allowed to take positions however they are the most comfortable.

Another set of folk recommendations regarding labor involves herbs or edibles to ease the labor process. The most feared aspect of labor is that it is painful, and women have sought help in making the experience less so. Various substances have been described since antiquity to help with pain in general, from alcohol to opium. But no present-day birth attendants are recommending that women take swigs of gin or smoke a hash pipe to feel better. Two herbs still occasionally mentioned as helping with labor pains are mugwort and wormwood, the latter of which is used to make absinthe. The association between these herbs and childbirth may go back to when they were first named. Both plants belong to the genus *Artemisia*, named for the Greek goddess Artemis, who was thought to preside over childbirth.[7] Artemis herself was a virgin and the goddess of chastity, but she was thought to be helpful for women in labor because she caused her mother, Leto, no pain during her delivery. She is also said to have helped her mother get through the birth of her brother, Apollo. Herbalists in past centuries are noted to have used these plants, especially wormwood, for assistance with difficult and painful births. Interestingly, these plants have been used medicinally for parturition in Southeast Asia as well, where no one has even heard of Artemis.[8]

Another plant that is said to help with childbirth is the date. This fruit is native to the Middle East, where the instructions for use in labor originate. Date juice was mentioned as a labor remedy in ancient Egyptian papyri from thousands of years ago.[9] It is also mentioned in the Quran, the holy book of Islam, and its account of Jesus's birth. What many people do not realize is that Mary, the mother of Jesus, is revered in Islam, and her name is mentioned more often in the Quran than in the entire New Testament. In Sura 19 of the Quran, Mary is described as suffering from the pains of childbirth. In her anguish, she gripped the trunk of a palm tree and cried out. A heavenly voice answered her, stating, "And shake toward you the trunk of the palm tree; it will drop upon you ripe, fresh dates."[10] Although it never explicitly states that the dates were meant to ease labor pain, one can see how a reader would make that connection.

It is easy to see that dates may provide a nourishing snack during labor, but could dates actually improve the labor experience? A group of Jordanian researchers decided to find out.[11] They studied a group of 114 women in their final month of pregnancy. Half of the women were given dates and told to eat six pieces a day until labor began. The other half were told to avoid dates for the rest of the pregnancy. While pain was not directly measured, the women who had eaten dates were noted to have shorter labors, particularly in the first part or "latent phase" when cervical dilation occurs more slowly. They were also more likely to go into spontaneous labor and less likely to need medicine to augment or strengthen their labor pains. It remains to be seen whether dates may really be a useful prescription for women looking to have an easy labor, but the study suggests that they may have some benefit.

The red raspberry leaf is also frequently mentioned as being helpful in labor. The raspberry leaf has been used medicinally since at least the sixth century. A 1941 article from the British medical journal *The Lancet* calls it "the best known and oldest of all the herb infusions and [is] included as a proved aid in maternity in the most ancient of herbal books."[12] More recently, there has been renewed medical interest in whether it may actually be helpful in the labor setting. A clinical trial randomly assigned women having their first baby to either take a pill containing raspberry leaf extract or placebo through the last two months of pregnancy.[13] Sad to say, there was no difference in pain or labor length for the women using this remedy. The only difference was that women who used the raspberry extract did not have to push for as long, but the difference was only ten minutes. On the other hand, there were no harmful effects either. So even though the ancient herbalists were wrong on this one, there would be no harm in a cup of raspberry leaf tea prior to labor.

In fact, teas and infusions have been a common theme in folk remedies for women in labor. Native American tribes have recommended teas made from certain herbs, or simply drinking lots of hot water during labor.[14] A less appealing beverage is the brew that Pliny the Elder wrote about in his tract *Naturalis Historia*, mixing powdered sows' dung with water to ensure an easy labor.[15] Another unsavory tea is recommended by certain Indian women for a labor that is not progressing; they instruct the laboring woman to drink water in which her mother-in-law soaked her big toe.[16] Though too bizarre (and downright disgusting) for common use, there is a pattern in many recommendations for women to drink tall glasses of water or tea during labor.

This set of instructions is quite different from what most laboring women hear from their doctors, which is not to eat or drink anything in labor. This advice is based on the concern that a few women will experience an emergency so dire that general anesthesia is required for rapid delivery. With general anesthesia, it is necessary to place a tube in the woman's throat to help her breathe, and if the stomach is full of fluid then there is a risk that fluid can be inhaled when the tube is inserted, causing a serious lung infection. Although this is a rare event, the outcome is serious enough that laboring women are advised not to take the risk and to keep the stomach empty throughout labor. Drinking might also be discouraged in labor because many doctors think it will slow down contractions. It is common practice for physicians to advise women experiencing preterm contractions to drink lots of fluid, since women who are dehydrated tend to have more frequent and stronger contractions. In this case, the doctors' advice is quite the opposite of the old wives who push for increasing fluids in labor.

Which advice is more valid? There are not many studies that measure how much liquid women drink in labor. However, in studies that compare slower rates of intravenous fluid drip with faster rates, labor is significantly shorter in the women who get more fluid.[17] Among women who were allowed to drink in labor, the ones who were also given additional intravenous hydration had shorter labors. One study demonstrated that women allowed to keep drinking during their labors had higher rates of vomiting, but again showed shorter labor lengths among women who had the most intravenous fluid hydration.[18] Obviously for the ancients, intravenous administration of fluid was not an option. But no matter what vile additive was placed in the beverage, the idea of providing sufficient fluid refreshment to the laboring mother does seem to have merit.

Encouraging women to relax during childbirth is another theme of labor folklore. Noticing that women who had difficult labors were sweaty and tense, while women with easy labors were more steady and relaxed, many birth attendants thought that the pain of labor could be eased by having the woman take steps to calm herself. Of course, whether staying calm is a cause or an effect of easy labor is a matter for debate. A woman having a difficult labor is likely to have more pain and become tenser due to the length and intensity of her labor; her tenseness does not necessarily increase the labor pain. Nevertheless, many forms of relaxation, including massage and the creation of a soothing environment, have been touted.

Early Mesopotamian writings recommend massaging the mother's belly while rubbing in a medicinal salve mixed with oil from the top to the bottom seven times.[19] Several cultures, including ones in Southeast

Asia, Brazil, and Central America, advocate massaging the laboring mother's abdomen, back, or legs to relax her and improve the quality of labor. Often, the recommendation for massage involves the vaginal opening itself. In this case, the goal is probably not so much to relax the mother as it is to use a form of lubrication. Various oils have been recommended, probably with the concept that making the exit for the baby slippery will help it to come out a bit faster. Ancient Romans advocated the liberal use of warm olive oil for this purpose. An ancient Greek recommendation involved fumigating the vagina with the fat of a hyena.[20] The olive oil seems a lot more pleasant.

This practice is echoed today when women may be instructed by their caregivers to massage the perineum. Perineal massage with oil or other lubricants is a common practice thought to help the vaginal opening to stretch. The intention is not necessarily to make labor easier. Rather it is to prevent tearing and the need for stitches. Several studies have suggested that perineal massage, or even just the application of a warm compress to the perineum in labor, can prevent injury.[21] So even if it doesn't make the labor shorter or less painful, massage of the vulva may be useful.

Other techniques that have been recommended for relaxation include playing soothing music, laboring by a riverside (or in more recent times, underwater), inhaling sweet-smelling fragrances, or applying heat to the belly or back.[22] In the late eighteenth century, a more startling tool for relaxation was in vogue. Early obstetricians noted that bloodletting seemed to lessen the pain of childbirth. William Dewees, an author of one of the most prominent textbooks of the time, wrote that draining a woman's blood was very helpful in improving pain and shortening difficult labors.[23] He wrote that the quick and easy labors that he observed "could be from no other cause than relaxation, produced by alarming haemorrhagy." It is not difficult to imagine that a profoundly anemic woman may indeed become "relaxed," since she would be so weak and faint that she could hardly move. This practice fortunately did not last, since it would put both the mother's health as well as the health of her baby at serious risk.

The dangers of this approach explain why it did not last the century. Many other recommendations about how to relax in labor continue to be discussed in the twenty-first century. In addition to massage, women may be told to try hypnotherapy, yoga, and mind-body techniques such as meditation and visualization.[24] Many of these therapies have been studied in the medical literature to see if there truly is an effect in improving pain or shortening labor.[25] Evaluating these studies has to be approached with a bit of skepticism about the conclusions. Women who enroll in studies of nonpharmacological treatments for pain, or who allow themselves to be randomly assigned to receive such a treatment or placebo, are likely to be more receptive to controlling pain without drugs. Since researchers usually rate the success of these treatments based on how satisfied a woman is with her labor, or how many drugs she used along the way, it may not be appropriate to say that a successful result means that all women will find it successful. A woman who wants or expects medicine for pain relief during labor will give a very different answer about how satisfied she was. Furthermore, there is considerable variation in how such therapies are practiced and taught. Nevertheless, some benefits have been demonstrated.

Studies that specifically look at relaxation techniques have shown that they do reduce pain intensity and increase satisfaction with pain relief.[26] In one trial, yoga proved not only to reduce pain, but also to shorten the overall length of labor when compared to usual care. A single controlled trial of massage therapy in labor demonstrated reduced pain and anxiety in the women who used it. In five trials, women who were taught self-hypnosis had less need for pain medicine and epidural anesthesia. Women relying only on aromatherapy or listening to relaxing music did not have any demonstrable improvement in their pain experience. None of these interventions are likely to have the kind of profound effect on pain provided by anesthetics that are injected or inhaled. Nevertheless, the evidence suggests that relaxation therapies can improve the labor experience for women who wish to avoid medical interventions or drugs in labor.

Perhaps no technique is as relaxing and soothing as having someone there to give the laboring woman encouragement, support, and reassurance. The so-called support person has been a fixture in labor scenes throughout history. Any artwork that depicts a laboring woman shows her with an attendant, usually female, who is holding her or standing beside her, giving both physical and emotional support. The expectation that a woman will have someone helping her through the labor process is not necessarily folklore in the purest sense, but it is a practice that seems universal in its description across different cultures and historical time periods. It is also one that is supported by medical science. There is robust evidence that women who have a continuous support person in labor to provide one-on-one assistance are more likely to have shorter labors and less likely to need surgical deliveries.[27] There is even some evidence that their babies are less likely to have difficulty at birth. The medical reasoning behind this phenomenon is that the constant encouragement and support reduces anxiety, which may reduce stress hormones that can have a harmful effect on labor. Although many women hope that a spouse, a significant other, or a helpful labor floor nurse will provide that kind of help, many look elsewhere and may even hire a woman trained specifically in labor support. Whatever the source of comfort, having a continuous support person is a great boon in labor and is one of the most effective recommendations for improving the labor experience.

A final piece of folklore surrounding labor stems from the observation that women who work hard during pregnancy seem to have easier and faster labors. This observation was recorded by midwives in the seventeenth century, who noted that having an easy pregnancy meant a difficult delivery, and vice versa.[28] They encouraged women to engage in hard toil while pregnant in order to facilitate delivery. This recommendation lies in contrast to many medical voices of later textbooks, who viewed the pregnant woman as a delicate being who needed to avoid taxing herself to ensure a safe pregnancy. Even into the twentieth century, however, women recorded folk beliefs about how hard work will yield an easy birth. One collection that summarized the beliefs of women in a California clinic included quotations such as, "Keep working and exercise. That makes an easier time in labor," and "If you work hard, labor is easier because women in Europe do that."[29] In fact, this observation has been made in several cultures. One nineteenth-century anthropologist who spent time touring the underdeveloped areas of Africa and Asia noted that women who worked throughout pregnancy in these lands had easier labors, and labor was notably "worse with those who idle beforehand."[30]

It is difficult to say just how much hard work has an effect on the labor experience, since different forms of employment involve such different amounts of activity and movement. A woman who sits at a desk all day for her job may feel like she is working very hard, but is having a very different experience from a woman tilling the soil on her farm all day. A reasonable substitute to asking "How hard do you work?" would be to measure the amount of aerobic activity or exercise that a woman practices, which may give a sense of how often and how strenuous activity during pregnancy may be. While many studies have examined the benefits of exercise on maternal health and fetal well-being, there are also a few that comment on how it affects labor.

One study that looked at women having a first baby found that those who participated in aerobic exercise at least three times weekly throughout the first and second trimester were half as likely to have a Cesarean section as those who did not.[31] After adjusting for other factors such as weight gain and use of epidural, the researchers found that nonexercisers were 4.5 times more likely to undergo Cesarean delivery. In a paper that combined the results of many other studies that compared women who exercised in pregnancy and those who did not, the authors confirmed a significant reduction in the risk of having a Cesarean section in women who exercised regularly.[32] There was not enough information from these trials about the length of labor to comment on whether aerobic activity could affect how long women spent in childbirth. Still, the science suggests that regular aerobic activity in pregnancy, whether through exercise or work, may have benefits on the course of labor.

Despite the favorable outcomes for women who follow some of these recommendations, no one promises labor is going to be easy. The hard fact remains that human childbirth involves a baby squeezing through a sensitive and narrow opening, and it involves pain. Most women in developed nations choose to give birth in hospitals, where treatments and medications can be used to make the birth less painful and to make sure the mother and baby remain as healthy as possible. But it is reassuring to know that some of their elders' advice may be helpful as well. Working hard in pregnancy may pay off in an easier labor, and maybe a little snack of dates can provide some energy to deal with the strain. Most importantly, the strongest benefits are likely to be had from doing whatever it takes to relax and be reassured that everything is going to be okay.

10

AFTER BIRTH

At last, nine months of pregnancy and many hours of labor are over. The new mother finally gets to hold her newborn child, thankful for all the advice and help she received to get to this thrilling moment. Many women at this point would think, "Mission accomplished!" and be done with listening to the opinions of well-meaning friends and Internet "experts." But there is still much folklore associated with the period immediately following delivery.

Some of this lore concerns the placenta, a source of fascination for women across the centuries. Although the function of the placenta is well known to most people who have taken a high school biology class, its purpose is not obvious to someone who doesn't understand basic physiology. Its appearance is also nothing like any other waste product that gets expelled from the human body. It's easy to see why the placenta would be a mystery to a member of a primitive culture. A birth attendant's knowledge about the placenta would be based on the three things that she would observe. It is a structure that always comes out after the infant appears. It is always attached to the baby by the umbilical cord, but not for very long, and it can be removed without injury to the baby. And even though it comes from the mother, it does not seem to be a part of her and she gets along fine afterward without it. Based on these observations, many cultures see the placenta as a structure that is somehow spiritually or organically linked to the health of the child. Some cultures literally view the placenta as a twin of the child, or as a sort of companion that escorts the infant into the world. Many rituals have been described that arise from this sort of belief.[1]

The most common ritual that is observed in preindustrial cultures is the burial of the placenta. This rite is performed to demonstrate respect for the placental "being," as one would for any member of the community. However, the placenta is often seen as having an influence on the child, and so burial rituals may be imbued with a sense of sympathetic magic. In other words, practitioners believe that what happens to the placenta can in some way influence the life of the child. The burial may be performed for the protection of the child, for example, as protection from evil spirits, or by figuratively "grounding" the child so its soul will not leave this world. Burial may also establish a connection between the child and the community (as with a burial in a specific tribal land). Treatment of the placenta is also seen as conferring attributes on the child. For example, burying the placenta near water may ensure that the child will be a good swimmer, or burying it under a fruit tree would endow the child with future fertility. Some cultures have an even more intricate association between the placenta and trees and encourage the mother to hang the placenta from a tree, whose health is then tied together with the infant's well-being.

There are very few women in today's Western society who share these beliefs or go looking to take their placentas home for a proper burial. No pregnancy websites are recommending that women should hang their placentas from the tree outside the kitchen window. A newer form of folklore regarding the placenta, however, has become increasingly pervasive in the past few decades. Some women are being encouraged by their friends, doulas, or midwives to eat the placenta following birth. The proponents of eating the placenta claim that it may have various health benefits. Most commonly, they recommend doing so to feel more energetic and recover quickly, to prevent postpartum depression, or to improve the milk supply and lead to better breastfeeding.[2]

Unlike other pieces of folklore discussed in this book, there are no significant precedents for this practice in human history. The most common reason that women give for following this advice is not that it was practiced by previous generations, but instead that it is seen as a behavior among other species of mammal. Since consumption of the placenta goes on in the natural world, the thinking goes, it must be natural and healthy for human mothers to do so as well. In fact, lower mammals are thought to eat the placenta mostly as a matter of safety because leaving the placenta behind may attract predators who will sense that there are young and defenseless newborns nearby who would make a tasty meal. Although one study suggested that eating the placenta may confer some relief from pain in rodents, there is no scientific evidence to suggest that this effect is duplicated in humans. [3]

Medicinal properties have been ascribed to the placenta since ancient times. A sixteenth-century compendium of Chinese medicine includes human placenta as an ingredient in a remedy for exhaustion and anemia. Certain cultures have recommended placenta as a cure for epilepsy or seizures. It has also been used in various forms both to promote fertility and to prevent pregnancy. However, all of these recommendations involve using the placenta as an ingredient in medicines for others, and not for the mother to consume her own placenta.

The advice for women to eat their own placentas following birth (officially referred to as placentophagy) seems to be a modern concept with few historical references. A physician writing nearly one hundred years ago mentioned hearing a superstition involving making a placental soup to improve milk production. [4] A paper from the 1970s that first noted the practice in the American counterculture reported that this behavior was also seen in some areas of Vietnam. [5] The only biblical reference to placentophagy comes in Deuteronomy (28:55–57). The passage describes what will happen to the Israelites if they do not follow the laws of God. Following a long litany of curses (pestilence, drought, madness, etc.), the Bible elaborates what will happen to women after their cities are besieged by enemies. They are starved and so hungry that "the tender and delicate woman among you" will be set against "her afterbirth that cometh out from between her feet, and against her children whom she shall bear, for she shall eat them for want of all things secretly in the siege." In other words, their hunger will be so dire that they will engage in cannibalism and placentophagy just to live. The implication is that if people do not follow God's orders, He will reduce them to the level of beasts. There is no suggestion of a benefit other than perhaps the nutritional value for someone who is dying of starvation.

Nevertheless, there has been a recent surge in the popularity of placentophagy, either as a dish cooked for a postpartum meal, or as an encapsulated medication taken for a period of time following birth.

While there have been no studies directly comparing the use of these capsules with placebo, there has not been any demonstrated benefit of taking placental supplements on either the prevention of postpartum depression or on the improvement of breastfeeding. An article that reviewed all of the medical studies that have looked at placental consumption concluded that, based on the limited information we have currently, there is no medical benefit to eating one's placenta, and the risks are uncertain.[6]

Following the expulsion of the placenta, the birth process is completed, and the exhausted mother now has the opportunity to rest and recover from her obstetrical ordeal. How long she should take to recover, and what steps she should take to hasten her recovery, are other frequently debated topics between women eager to provide advice.

Nearly every culture in the world has some form of a prescribed recovery ritual. After what may be hours of labor pain, physical exhaustion of pushing the baby out, and actual trauma to sensitive perineal tissues that have torn and stretched, it is clear that time is needed for physical recovery. In some cultures, pregnancy and delivery are viewed as a disease state that requires time for reversal of its effects. For some, the delivery process is viewed as "unclean," particularly due to the amount of bleeding involved and the persistence of bleeding for weeks thereafter. Postpartum recovery rituals may be cleansing or restorative, allowing the mother to reenter society when she regains her normal stature. Finally, the postpartum recovery phase may be seen as a period of bonding, when the mother is allowed uninterrupted time to nurture and feed her baby.

Remarkably, the amount of time reserved for postpartum recovery is fairly consistent between cultures and across continents. Nearly all cultures recommend a resting period of thirty to forty days. In China and Southeast Asian countries,[7] activity is limited for one month. In India,[8] Turkey,[9] and the Middle East,[10] the length of time is specified as forty days. This is also the length of time prescribed by Native Americans in the American Southwest.[11] Even in a Bedouin community where society is nomadic and families may be frequently on the move, the recommendation for limiting activity after delivery is forty days.[12]

In the Christian church, there is a tradition that also coincides with the forty-day rule. "Churching of Women" is a liturgical rite in which new mothers are invited to return to church on the fortieth day following delivery, both as a form of spiritual cleansing and as a way to rejoin the community.[13] The tradition dates back to the very early days of Christianity, and follows the example set by Mary when she presented to the temple to fill the requirements of the Laws of Moses (Luke 2:22). Although few modern congregants engage in this rite, there are still areas, particularly in Eastern Orthodoxy, where it is followed.

Nowadays, medical traditions still keep the recovery period at about forty days. In many Western nations, women are given the opportunity to take maternity leave for up to six months, but the period of time described by physicians as needed for physical recovery is generally standardized at six weeks. This amount of time, often referred to as the "puerperium," is about how long it takes for the uterus to reach its normal nonpregnant size and all of the pregnancy changes in the body to return to normal.

Although various cultures agree that this four- to six-week time span is needed for recovery, the restrictions prescribed often seem drastic. Although rest is universally recommended and most authorities advise women against performing housework and chores, women are often encouraged to remain in bed for long periods of time. In China and Vietnam, resting in bed is encouraged as much as possible, and in Bangladesh and Turkey, women are confined to the house in seclusion. A nineteenth-century American textbook on obstetrics made the following recommendation for new mothers:

> The woman's stay in bed . . . should be absolute for the first six days. . . . Thereafter the bed should be changed every two to three days. She should remain in bed at least three weeks, oftener longer, than less. . . . Only at the end of the thirtieth day will we allow her to walk. . . . She should not venture out before the sixth week.[14]

Although such advice was commonly given at one time, it is now recognized that such extreme restriction is not only unwarranted, but may actually be harmful. Prolonged bed rest puts women at increased risk of medical complications such as blood clots in the legs or pneumonia. For most women, health care providers now encourage walking and fresh air as soon as possible after birth.

In China, women engage in a highly regimented practice following delivery that is called *zuoyuezi*, or "doing the month."[15] This tradition, which dates back to the Song dynasty of the eleventh to twelfth century, involves a group of recommendations intended to restore balance to the mother's health and help her recover from the trauma of childbirth. In addition to restriction of activity (which includes resting in bed for most of the day), *zuoyuezi* involves following a special diet that is rich in foods such as egg, chicken, animal viscera, soup, bean curd, and rice. Women are also restricted from bathing and washing hair in order to avoid exposure to cold, which is felt to be harmful.

Recently, a study was performed to examine the effect of following this regimen.[16] Researchers surveyed 198 Chinese women in order to compare the experiences of those who followed this regimen with those who did not. The authors assessed the women six weeks after delivery and measured their endurance and muscle strength, as well as their physical and mood symptoms. The degree to which women followed the prescribed practices was highly variable, but 40 percent of women remained supine most or all of the time, and 47 percent did not take a bath during that time. Adherence to "doing the month" was significantly correlated with poor walking endurance and increased depressive symptoms. The authors conclude that following a course of activity restriction in the postpartum period may actually worsen both physical and mental health.

As for how soon a woman can return to work safely or resume a baseline level of activity, there is very little true research. The Departments of Health in several countries have guidelines as to when women may return to normal activity, but they are generally worded vaguely.[17] For example, the U.S. guidelines suggest that women can return to prepregnancy routines "gradually as soon as it is physically and medically safe." In the United Kingdom, the guidelines state that mild exercise may begin immediately if the pregnancy and delivery were uncomplicated. Unfortunately, there is no reliable research to dictate exactly when it is safe to resume work, and this issue is dependent on so many related factors, including preexisting health, work and family commitments, and availability of social support.[18] In this case, a woman should probably rely on her best judgment over the opinion of others' advice.

Another aspect of postpartum recovery for which many women seek advice is how soon they can resume having sex. Many of the folk traditions from other cultures that restrict postpartum activity specifically ban any vaginal intercourse while the woman is recovering. Most frequently, these recommendations are made out of concern for the mother's health. For example, women fear that vaginal penetration may cause or worsen tearing of the vagina, or increase the chance that the womb's attachments will loosen and the uterus will prolapse. Sometimes the concern is the impurity of the mother, which is only lifted when the postpartum bleeding and discharge stop completely. For example, in Zimbabwe men are told that if they have sex with a woman who is still bleeding, he will suffer from "musana," an illness featuring backache and dysfunction of his sex organ.[19] Of course, this may be an invention of the women in that culture who wished to avoid early intercourse; to cover all bases, men are also told that if they have sex with another woman during this time, it will cause their child to become ill.

In Western medicine, it has become common for obstetric providers to routinely advise women not to have sex for at least six weeks. They voice concern about the risk of infection by possibly introducing bacteria into the uterus and also of injuring areas that might have torn during the birth process. Evidence demonstrates that intercourse may actually be safe earlier than that, provided the mother feels she is ready. About half of women are sexually active before they have their six-week postpartum appointment, though it depends heavily on the route of delivery, the age of the patient, and how sexually active she was at the beginning of pregnancy.[20] The American College of Obstetrics and Gynecology guidelines state that the risk of bleeding and infection are minimal after the first two weeks. Another study suggested that even in cases where women had episiotomies (that is, having been cut to make extra room at the time of birth), there is enough healing by the third week for intercourse to occur without further harm.[21]

Clearly there are many other reasons to avoid intercourse, and women who are still sore, sleepless, and stressed from having a newborn may feel that sex is the farthest thing from their minds. But it is yet another example of where some old wives' advice may be a bit inaccurate.

The recommendations that deal with postpartum recovery are mostly born out of concern for the mother's well-being. There is a general acknowledgment that recovering from a vaginal birth can be a difficult time, and so these pieces of folklore urge women to take the time they need to feel better and fully functional in taking care of their babies. How much they are followed will depend on each woman's health and birth experience, but ultimately she must use her common sense to decide how seriously to take these recommendations.

11

BREASTFEEDING

For a process that seems as though it should be so instinctive and natural, breastfeeding generates a lot of anguish and confusion. Breasts start to produce milk immediately after birth occurs, and infants are hardwired from birth to suck on the nipple to get their nutrition. And yet many women have difficulty with the process, either because the amount of milk produced isn't enough, or because the baby has difficulty with latching on. Difficulties with breastfeeding have made lactation one of the richest areas in folklore and folk advice. Women from all walks of life who have been through the process are eager to share their experiences and give new mothers recommendations about how to overcome breastfeeding difficulties.

The folklore on breastfeeding doesn't just come from family and friends. Even lactation consultants, who are specially trained in breast-feeding issues in order to educate others, pass on some unusual advice. In 1974, a member of La Leche League International, an organization that supports breastfeeding and education about lactation, asked her colleagues about the superstitions and old wives' tales they had heard about.[1] She described all manner of tips that her fellow consultants were familiar with, and many that they believed were useful and recommended. The advice covered various aspects of breastfeeding, including ways to enhance milk supply, getting milk to dry up, aiding sore breasts or nipples, and avoiding foods that could interfere with breastfeeding.

In the forty years since then, the science of lactation has become more developed, with professional organizations and journals devoting considerable time and resources to studying best practices for breast-feeding. The folk remedies that were mentioned forty years earlier, though, are still being discussed among experts in the field. A recent survey of lactation educators that was conducted online in the United States demonstrated that 69 percent of specialists surveyed were aware of traditional folk remedies, and many of them continued to recommend such practices to their clients.[2] The most commonly recommended remedies fall into the categories of promoting lactation, reducing pain associated with breastfeeding, and avoiding substances with adverse effects on the infant.

Advice for increasing milk production is heard most often. Not producing enough breast milk can be a troubling and anxiety-provoking problem for many new mothers. Not only is there the risk for the infant of inadequate nutrition and dehydration, but many women see it as a personal failure for which they take responsibility. Remedies rumored to increase the production of breast milk are frequently sought to help women overcome this perceived failing. Most of the recommendations in this category involve eating or drinking some nutritional supplement that will boost the milk supply. For example, dairy cattle are often fed alfalfa to improve their milk production, so women are encouraged to try the same. Some recommendations involve a bit more work. A recommendation from Sri Lanka, for example, advises women to hang the placenta from a fig tree to promote milk production. This folklore demonstrates an interesting combination of themes: the placenta being tied to the baby's health and well-being, the fig tree having many seeds reminiscent of fertility, and the branches of the tree representing some relationship to the sustenance of life.

In terms of supplemental foodstuffs, the one that is most frequently recommended for boosting the milk supply is beer. New mothers were often told to drink beer by physicians in the late nineteenth century, with several medical texts suggesting that it may help a mother to improve nursing. One such text specifically recommends "porter or ale taken once or twice a day" to promote the secretion of milk.[3] In the early 1900s, beer companies would even market low alcohol beers to new mothers for the purpose of increasing their strength and enhancing their yield of milk.[4] The practice may date as far back as ancient Egypt, since there is a citation in the Ebers papyrus that mentions a reed rubbed in sweet beer to improve a mother's milk supply.[5] One authority in the Babylonian Talmud (from the third century), however, cautions that hops are injurious to milk, but wine will increase the amount of milk.[6]

Alcohol was used as a cure for a lot of problems in past centuries, and it was likely to help with anything where intoxication would take someone's mind off her problem. In the last century, the dangers of alcohol to mothers and babies were more widely recognized, and fewer and fewer medical sources encouraged mothers to drink alcohol. Still, with the persistence of women recommending beer as a helpful agent, some researchers have explored the question of whether it really could improve milk production. But studies have shown that maternal alcohol consumption can actually decrease milk production,[7] and that infants exposed to milk of women who have been drinking alcohol will spend less time at the breast, perhaps because of an unpleasant taste that the alcohol gives to breast milk.[8]

However, there is some evidence that beer might actually be of some help to nursing mothers, but not necessarily due to alcohol. Some studies show that drinking beer can cause a rise in the level of prolactin, a pituitary hormone that stimulates the breast to make milk. Prolactin levels have been shown to increase after drinking beer in women who were not breastfeeding; this was also true for men. In a study where alcoholic and nonalcoholic varieties of beer were compared, the prolactin levels increased the same amount in both groups. When these women were given plain alcohol, the prolactin level did not rise.[9] This would suggest something unique about beer that could influence prolactin secretion.

Several ingredients of beer have been examined, though mostly in experiments done on animals.[10] Rats that were fed either a powder made from dehydrated beer or an extract that was made from barley had similar changes in prolactin levels. Sheep exposed to different components showed the prolactin response when they were given barley or crude malt, but not when given an extract made from hops, another plant used in brewing beer. The evidence would suggest that this hormone is promoted by some component of the barley that is used for brewing and does not require any alcohol to be present. Although there have been no studies that definitively prove a beneficial effect of nonalcoholic beer, there is likely no harm in trying it, particularly if one has a taste for beer without alcohol.

If indeed barley is helpful in promoting milk production, it may explain the use of other grains by mothers interested in improving their milk supply. Various herbs and grains have been recommended by authorities in the past. There is probably some association made between milk production in cows, who graze on various crops, and the power of these grains to cause similar effects in lactating women. Alfalfa, as mentioned previously, is a commonly recommended grain that is said to improve the milk supply. The Trotula, a medieval compendium of early pharmacology and herbal remedies for women, recommends a diet of porridge made from beans, rice, and wheat to help the breastfeeding mother.[11] Oatmeal is a remedy mentioned in many cultures, and a physician writing in the nineteenth century supported its use based on his personal experience with his patients who used it.[12] All of these grains sound healthy, and there would be no arguments from doctors in letting new mothers have a bowl of cereal. However, no studies have shown that any grains specifically improve milk production.

An herb that is commonly mentioned as promoting milk production is silymarin, which is familiarly known as milk thistle. In the previously mentioned survey of modern lactation consultants, 23 percent of respondents recommended this herb.[13] It may be that its reputation for use by breastfeeding moms is based on the name, "milk thistle." This label, however, has nothing to do with its effect on lactation. Instead, it got the name because when the leaves are crushed, they release a milky white sap that is reminiscent of breast milk. This may be yet another example of folklore that is based on an association between two things that look alike. For whatever reason that some women began to use it for this purpose, this herb may actually have a beneficial effect on milk production. In the only clinical trial that looked at using this herb,[14] fifty women were divided into two groups: one that took a silymarin extract and the other that took an identical placebo. After two months, the silymarin group had an 86 percent increase in the volume of milk produced, and the placebo group had a 32 percent increase. Not much is known about the long-term effects or safety of using milk thistle, but such a result suggests that more study about using this herb is warranted.

Perhaps the most popular herbal remedy cited for the promotion of breastfeeding is fenugreek. Fenugreek is an herb that has been prescribed since antiquity for various uses, but it is unclear when the link to breastfeeding was established.[15] The ancient Greek herbalist Dioscorides mentioned it as early as the first century BCE as having a beneficial effect in recovery from childbirth. Other ancient texts mention it as a useful additive to fodder for oxen and cattle.[16] Perhaps a combination of these associations led women to try it for breastfeeding. In any case, the first citation of its use for this reason in medical literature was not until 1945. Since then there have been an overwhelming number of anecdotal reports that support its use, with women who take fenugreek saying that they see an improvement in breast milk production within one to three days. There has been only one scientifically conducted clinical trial that showed a positive effect, which required that women take two to three tablets three times daily.[17] Although there may be a benefit, there is also some risk with such large doses of this herb. It may cause diarrhea and can trigger worsening of asthma in women with this disease. Even so, it may be a successful remedy for women who feel they need to make a little more milk to nourish their babies.

Another common problem that women face is the soreness and discomfort that goes along with breastfeeding. Painful breasts may be a result of engorgement, when the breast ducts swell in the days following delivery as the milk "comes in." Pain may also come in the form of sore nipples, due to the vigorous sucking of the infant before the mother is used to it. In either case, the discomfort is usually limited to a few days, and it will go away on its own. The breast ducts grow to accommodate the increased volume of fluid that comes with lactation, and the pain from being swollen subsides. As babies nurse in the first few weeks, the skin of the nipples toughens and is less likely to become raw or cracked. Nevertheless, such pain can be sufficiently troublesome to provoke women to seek methods of relief.

Since engorgement is associated with a sudden increase in fluid, treatments may be recommended that reduce the volume of fluid. Many authors have quite sensibly recommended that the best approach to reducing engorgement is to have the infant suckle frequently and for enough time to empty out the swollen breast ducts. Centuries ago, doctors had other ideas about how to get fluid out of body extremities. A common remedy for all sorts of swelling was leeches, and they were seen as suitable for relieving breast swelling as well. A medical textbook written as late as the early nineteenth century advised applying leeches to the bottom aspect of the breast to relieve "milk fever."[18] Fortunately, such advice is a thing of the past, and no old wives tell women to place parasites on their breasts anymore.

Other remedies to soothe breast discomfort that are still in vogue involve placing less disgusting objects on the breast. Traditional medicine often recommends that pain be relieved by applying a poultice, which is typically described as a mass of cloth with herbs or liquid meant to drape over the offending organ. In the case of the breast, several suggestions have been made for poultices that would cover the area. The French have suggested applying a warm pancake or omelet to the breast to relieve its swelling.[19] One of the most common suggestions has been the use of cabbage leaves. The most likely explanation for this particular remedy is the shape of the leaves, which conform well to the contour of the breast. Though most authorities recommend using it intact and applied to the surface of the breast, the French physician Francois Mauriceau mentioned using cabbage ground up into a poultice along with chamomile leaves.[20]

Using cabbage leaves to treat engorgement is still commonly mentioned in modern times. Several studies have been conducted to see if their use is helpful. One study demonstrated an improvement in breast pain when cabbage leaves were applied to the breast, but the effect was no different than simply applying a damp cloth to the breast.[21] In another study designed to see if the leaves could prevent pain, women were instructed to wear cabbage leaves on the breast before any pain or engorgement set in, but they had no effect in this case.[22] Other researchers have questioned whether certain qualities of cabbage may be helpful. In a study that compared the use of cooked cabbage leaves with raw ones, there was no difference in relief from pain.[23] The same group of researchers created a cream that contained cabbage leaf extract and compared the effect with a similar cream that did not contain cabbage.[24] Again, no difference was shown. After sifting through the many studies that have been done on cabbage leaves, a group of authors wrote a review that examined all of the available evidence on treatments for breast engorgement.[25] The authors concluded that there is no strong evidence for using cabbage leaves to help with engorgement.

Another sort of "compress" that has been advocated for use in soothing sore nipples is the tea bag. This remedy cannot have been around for too long since tea in prior centuries was prepared with free-floating leaves. Perhaps, though, there is some influence of historical experts such as Mauriceau who advocated the use of chamomile in soothing breast pain. Then again, it may have been used just because it is wet and floppy and clings to the surface of the breast. In any case, the tea bag is a widely available and easily prepared remedy that can be placed over a sore or cracked nipple.

This remedy, however, is not likely to be of much use. In one randomized trial, breastfeeding mothers who were assigned to use either tea bags, wet breast pads, or nothing rated the degree of soreness after the application. Although both tea bags and plain compresses were rated as more helpful than nothing, there was no difference between the two applications.[26] Another paper that reviewed several studies on the use of compresses to improve nipple pain concluded that using tea bags does not confer any benefit for the prevention or treatment of pain from breastfeeding.[27]

In summary, there is no particular folk remedy that appears to help with breastfeeding-related pain. Putting any kind of wet compress on the breast is probably helpful, the same way that placing a cool, wet rag on any sore body part will feel soothing. The most reliable factor to prevent or relieve pain from breastfeeding, though, is breastfeeding education that promotes proper positioning and timing of feedings.

Another common piece of advice offered to breastfeeding women has to do with what they are eating when they breastfeed. The composition of breast milk is pretty standard. Regardless of a woman's diet, culture, breast size, or background, the human breast produces the same liquid with concentrations of nutrients that will help her baby to thrive and grow. However, many women are told that what is in the breast milk will be affected by what they put in their stomachs. Such thinking again dates back many centuries. The medieval physician Aldobrandino of Siena warned women that ingesting foods with strong flavors such as onion, garlic, pepper, mint, and basil would cause milk to be too strong for the infant, who would then avoid suckling.[28] The Roman gynecologist Soranus also warned against leeks, onions, garlic, and radishes, as these would make the milk pungent.[29] The Trotula similarly cautions women to avoid leeks, onions, and pepper, "but above all garlic."[30]

In fact, a woman's diet may actually alter the taste of human milk. In one study, the flavor of milk was manipulated by feeding breastfeeding women capsules containing different flavors, such as banana, anise, and menthol.[31] There was significant variation in how long it took for each flavor to be detectable in the milk, and in how long the effect lingered. Even the most tenacious flavor (menthol) was gone at the end of eight hours, so these would not be expected to affect the baby's feeding for longer than that. Other studies have suggested that the flavor may indeed affect how long the baby suckles. But the Trotula had it wrong. The flavor of garlic actually made babies spend a longer time at the breast!

Another concern that women may hear about is the effect that their diet will have on the baby's digestion, and particularly on whether it can cause colic. Colic is a mysterious condition, where some otherwise healthy babies cry incessantly and can't be comforted. Although no one knows exactly what causes some babies to act this way, current thinking is that it is usually due to gastrointestinal distress, with the baby experiencing intestinal pain due to difficult digestion. Other babies may seem "gassy," with frequent noisy eruptions that don't seem to bother them but parents may find embarrassing when they are showing off their child. For the mothers, there are several foods that they may associate with their own indigestion or flatulence. All those childhood rhymes about beans are sung for a reason. In addition to beans, certain foods are known to increase gas production in the human gut, with cruciferous vegetables (like broccoli, cabbage, and brussels sprouts) being the big offenders. Could it be that mothers who eat a lot of these vegetables pass on some chemical in the breast milk that would make the baby more uncomfortable as well?

One study has addressed this issue by having breastfeeding women fill out a questionnaire about what foods they had consumed in the week prior to the study and what behaviors their infants exhibited during that time.[32] The authors reported that for women who had eaten more cruciferous vegetables, their babies were more likely to have symptoms of colic, even though they did not have other symptoms like diarrhea, constipation, or gassiness. Cow's milk and chocolate were also shown to have a small effect. Of note is that 61 percent of the women surveyed said they were told to avoid eating some of these foods by friends or colleagues. This confirms that this piece of folklore is being passed around liberally, and probably for good reason. There is, after all, a link between what the mother eats and how it affects her baby's behavior.

Overall, the body of folklore dealing with breastfeeding has quite a few examples of where the old wives got it right. Although the recommendations about cabbage leaves and tea bags are not justified, much of the advice passed down about improving milk supply and taking care to eat correctly are based in kernels of truth. Still, these are areas where there is not quite enough information to move them into the mainstream of medical recommendations. Even though herbs such as fenugreek or silymarin may improve milk supply, there is not enough information about maternal side effects and possible effects on exposed babies to recommend them for everyone. And even though one could make a good case for avoiding broccoli while breastfeeding, it may be unwise to restrict breastfeeding women from an entire class of otherwise healthy vegetables. Still, the fact that many of these pieces of advice have been borne out by scientific investigation makes a strong case for continued research on these old wives' tales.

12

AFTERTHOUGHTS AND CONCLUSIONS

From conception to weaning, the recommendations that get passed along from woman to woman are numerous and wide-ranging. Some of the advice is practical, like enjoying a soothing labor massage or applying a cool cabbage leaf to the sensitive breast. Other recommendations are just wacky. It is hard to imagine that anyone in modern society would seriously think that putting a knife under the labor bed or having sex lying on one's right side will actually have an effect on the pregnancy. Still, there are many suggestions that sound plausible, even if there is not a lot of hard evidence to prove their worth. We have seen that among the many old wives' tales discussed here, the old wives do not always know best, but there are many occasions where they make suggestions that are helpful.

The ones that are proven helpful, though, are a relatively small subset. Many of the traditional remedies mentioned here are based on magic and superstition and not on observing what really works. Performing masculine tasks to have a boy, opening locks to make an easy labor, eating milk thistle because it has a milky appearance—all of these are examples of "magical thinking," where the recommendation is expected to work only because it reminds the user of the result it is meant to achieve. This is a very different source from observation, where someone proposes a remedy because it seems to work, and then it works again the next time they use it. Observational study is a more reliable source of advice, and unfortunately, few of the traditional recommendations have been subjected to that kind of scrutiny.

The lack of scrutiny brings to mind another important point: this book is not an endorsement for any of these practices. I have provided examples of certain folklore that do seem to work, and some of these have a good amount of scientific research in support. However, every pregnancy is different, and what may be appropriate for one woman may not be appropriate for another. For example, even though castor oil or nipple stimulation may be helpful in inducing labor, it would be inappropriate for a woman at risk of premature labor to use either of these methods before she reaches full term. For pregnant women reading this book, I encourage you to consult your care provider to make sure it is safe before you follow any advice passed along by friends or relatives.

The list in this book is by no means exhaustive. There are plenty of tidbits passed along that I have not mentioned. One woman swears that she conceived boys every time she had sex in the afternoon. Another says that taking goat's rue was the secret to her bountiful milk production. No doubt there are hundreds of examples of folklore that may be passed around that were not included. Often these are remedies that are too obscure, having only been heard once or twice. The examples in this book are grouped together in patterns, where lots of similar recommendations are made in the same vein.

There are also many examples that were not included because they did not seem folkloric enough. Taking vitamins to conceive is based on modern medical concepts and not traditional thinking. Using hypnosis in labor is a form of relaxation, but not one that is likely to have been discussed for centuries. By its nature, folklore is fluid and changing, and perhaps such talk will seem traditional at some point down the road. Looking at the patterns of advice over time, though, is what this review was designed to accomplish.

Reviewing all of the advice that has been handed down through the ages, it is striking how many suggestions are still seen as relevant and possibly helpful. Even educated and well-informed women ask about induction methods and pregnancy diets that are reminiscent of what was written about hundreds of years ago. These same women would probably not show interest in other medical theories from the same era. Those ancient writers held some beliefs that today's scientists view as silly. For example, for those historical practitioners who had no concept of how blood circulated or how the immune system worked, health was seen as a balance of hot and cold humors. They expected sick people to get better through blood-letting that would allow harmful vapors to escape. Now that the human body is better understood, no one would take such a suggestion seriously. But when it comes to suggestions related to pregnancy, even the items mentioned in medical writings from pre-Christian times don't seem all that far-fetched. Telling the child's sex by evaluating the mother's urine, or boosting a mother's milk supply with a sip of beer were mentioned in Egyptian papyri from thousands of years ago. And here we are, still talking about them.

Of course, not everything mentioned in this book is that old. Trying to tell the baby's sex from the rate of its heartbeat is only as old as the stethoscope. Using pineapple to induce labor has only become more common after this fruit was widely available by shipping and exporting. Yet the sentiments behind them sound like what women of all centuries have heard as they tried to figure out how to have some control over their pregnancies.

Even though reviewing historical texts gives us some idea of what was understood by their authors, we don't really know what women in those times actually talked about regarding pregnancy. The information that we have from ancient times is relatively sparse. The information about biblical and Egyptian medicine is based on a handful of documents. Medical knowledge in ancient Greek and Roman times is gathered from a few dozen medical texts that have survived. Even with the advent of the printing press and the wide distribution of published books, very few books printed on paper survive more than a couple of centuries, since the bindings fall apart and the paper disintegrates. Those few texts on pregnancy really represent a tiny fraction of what has been written about this subject over the ages.

We know even less about the knowledge and opinions of women who helped with pregnancy and childbirth during this time. Medical texts and books have mostly been written by men. When medical men have been called to help with a birth or teach about pregnancy, it is usually for problems and diseases, when things go wrong. The women who were directly involved in attending childbirth were likely not in a position to be writing or teaching. They may not have been able to read at all. Their lore and knowledge about taking care of their pregnant sisters would have been passed on orally from one generation to the next. Maybe some of that knowledge is still being passed along and doesn't appear in any official medical or obstetrical writings.

Now we have entered an era different from any before. With the advent of the Internet, any woman can become an author. There has been an explosion of websites, chat rooms, and blogs where any woman can share her knowledge or opinions about pregnancy. The audience is no longer just the members of a local community, or the readers of a magazine, but anyone with access to a computer (sometimes referred to as "the blogosphere," an imagined world of eager readers!). At least in theory, any woman can share her experiences about pregnancy and her account of which remedies worked for her with anyone who will listen.

Ideally, all this advice would be shared responsibly and authoritatively. That is, such a woman would not tell other pregnant women to do anything that might be inherently dangerous to herself or her baby. The recommendations that would be shared would take into account that not every herb to be eaten is proven safe and not every activity is without risk. Also, these spreaders of information would back up their writings with some reliable evidence, even if it were anecdotal from personal experience. They wouldn't just pass along every item they hear without somehow checking if it would work.

Unfortunately, we don't live in an ideal world. Some Internet authors will offer advice that is neither safe nor sound. Likewise, there are many sites that offer products for sale that they claim have proven helpful effects, but really they are just trying to turn a profit with no such proof at hand. Not to say that these are common. There are many reputable sites out there that offer medical advice, or even nonmedical and traditional advice, by experienced and knowledgeable experts. The web-surfing pregnant lady, however, should approach her research with a healthy dose of skepticism and not be too gullible.

From a folkloric point of view, though, our era brings great potential for spreading information. Old wives tales may be passed along more completely and efficiently than ever before. Women of the next generation may have at their disposal not just the lore of sisters and friends, but of the female kinfolk of various cultures and geographical areas.

Hopefully, this explosion of lore will inspire more testing as well. Many of the research studies cited in this book were done simply because some scientist was curious about whether that remedy he kept hearing about was helpful or not. If it weren't for the advice of prior generations of womenfolk, would there have been studies on raspberry leaves or chasteberry? Would anyone have bothered to compare heartbeats and fetal gender? Research is often inspired by patterns that are noted by observation. Future scientists may hope that some of the links that have been observed by pregnant mothers are real, and they will find ways to test them.

For now, there are still plenty of observations to test. Science has greatly advanced our understanding of how pregnancy induces nausea, how labor starts, and how breast milk is produced. Even with all the increase in knowledge, though, we still don't know why women crave certain foods, or whether they can bring labor on with spicy food, or if herbal supplements can improve their milk supply. As much as such things can be tested, there will continue to be studies that explore the validity of such advice. Hopefully, soon there will be more complete answers to the questions raised by the old wives of yore.

NOTES

2. GETTING PREGNANT

1. Laszlo G. Jozsa, "Obesity in the Paleolithic era," *Hormones* 10 (2011): 241–44.

2. Harold Speert, *Obstetrics and Gynecology: A History and Iconography* (San Francisco: Norman Publishing, 1994), 409–54.

3. L. Rempelakos, Costas Tsiamis, and E. Poulakou-Rebelakou, "Penile representations in ancient Greek art," *Archivos Espanoles de Urologia* 66 (2013): 911–16.

4. Evangelos Spyropoulos et al., "Size of external genital organs and somatometric parameters among physically normal men younger than 40 years old," *Urology* 60 (2002): 485–89.

5. Grazyna Jasienska et al., "Large breasts and narrow waists indicate high reproductive potential in women," *Proceedings of the Royal Society of London B* 271 (2004): 1213–17.

6. Rosalind Franklin, *Baby Lore: Superstitions & Old Wives Tales from the World Over* (Sussex, UK: Diggory Press, 2005), 33–43.

7. Janet L. Sha, *Mothers of Thyme: Customs and Rituals of Infertility and Miscarriage* (Minneapolis: Lida Rose Press, 1990), 21–43.

8. Tamer Edirne et al., "Use of complementary and alternative medicines by a sample of Turkish women for infertility enhancement: a descriptive study," *BMC Complementary and Alternative Medicine* 10 (2010): 11–17.

9. Helen King, "Food as a symbol in classical Greece," *History Today* 36 (1986): 1–5.

10. Jorge E. Chavarro et al., "Diet and lifestyle in the prevention of ovulatory disorder infertility," *Obstetrics & Gynecology* 110 (2007): 1050–58.

11. Jorge E. Chavarro et al., "Use of multivitamins, intake of B vitamins, and risk of ovulatory infertility," *Fertility and Sterility* 89 (2008): 668–76.

12. Claudia Daniele et al., "Vitex agnus castus: a systematic review of adverse events," *Drug Safety* 28 (2005): 319–32.

13. Beatrix Roemheld-Hamm, "Chasteberry," *American Family Physician* 72 (2005): 821–24.

14. Lynn M. Westphal, Mary L. Polan, and Aileen S. Trant, "Double-blind, placebo-controlled study of Fertilityblend: a nutritional supplement for improving fertility in women," *Clinical Experiments in Obstetrics and Gynecology* 33 (2006): 205–8.

15. Beatrice Fontanel and Claire d'Harcourt, *Babies: History, Art and Folklore* (New York: Harry Abrams, 1997), 10–15.

16. Roy J. Levin, "The physiology of sexual arousal in the human female: a recreational and procreational synthesis," *Archives of Sexual Behavior* 31 (2002): 405–11.

17. Jacky Boivin et al., "The effects of female sexual response in coitus on early reproductive processes," *Journal of Behavioral Medicine* 15 (1992): 509–18.

18. Fontanel and d'Harcourt, *Babies*, 12.

19. Kaiyan Pei, Y. Xu, and Mengchun Jia, "Effect of successive ejaculation on semen analysis parameters in normal men," *Zhonghua Nan Ke Xue* 10 (2004): 667–70.

20. Nan B. Olderied, Hallgeir Rui, and Kenneth Purvis, "Life styles of men in barren couples and their relationship to sperm quality," *International Journal of Fertility* 37 (1992): 343–49.

21. Carolina H. J. Tiemessen, Johannes L. H. Evers, and Robert S. G. M. Bots, "Tight-fitting underwear and sperm quality," *Lancet* 347 (1996): 1844–45.

22. S. M. Matthiesen et al., "Stress, distress and outcome of assisted reproductive technology (ART): a meta-analysis," *Human Reproduction* 26 (2011): 2763–76.

23. Linda K. Bennington, "Can complementary and alternative medicine be used to treat infertility?" *MCN: The American Journal of Maternal/Child Nursing* 35 (2010): 140–47.

24. Ernest Hung Yu Ng et al., "The role of acupuncture in the management of subfertility," *Fertility and Sterility* 90 (2008): 1–13.

25. Speert, *Obstetrics and Gynecology*, 411.

26. Jonathan Schaffir, Alana McGee, and Elizabeth Kennard, "Use of nonmedical treatment by infertility patients," *Journal of Reproductive Medicine* 54 (2009): 415–20.

27. Robab Latifnejad Roudsari, Helen T. Allan, and Pam A. Smith, "Looking at infertility through the lens of religion and spirituality: a review of the literature," *Human Fertility* 10 (2007): 141–49.

28. Kwang Y. Cha, Daniel P. Wirth, and Rogerio A. Lobo, "Does prayer influence the success of in vitro fertilization-embryo transfer?" *Journal of Reproductive Medicine* 46 (2001): 781–87.

29. Bruce L. Flamm, "Prayer and the success of IVF," *Journal of Reproductive Medicine* 50 (2005): 71.

3. CHOOSING A BABY'S GENDER*

1. T. E. Page, "Regimen I, 27," in *Hippocrates*, vol. 4, translated by W. H. S. Jones (New York: Putnam, 1931).

2. Jonathan Schaffir, "What are little boys made of? The never-ending search for sex selection techniques," *Perspectives in Biology and Medicine* 34 (1991): 516–25.

3. Margaret Tallmadge May, *Galen: On the Usefulness of the Parts of the Body* (New York: Cornell University Press, 1968), 14:10.

4. Francois Mauriceau, *The Diseases of Women with Child, and in Childbed* (London: John Darby, 1683), 45–46.

5. Nicholas Culpeper, *A Directory for Midwives: Or, A Guide to Women in Their Conception, Bearing, and Suckling Their Children* (London: T. Norris, 1724).

6. Michael Thomas Sadler, *The Law of Population* (London: John Murray, 1830).

7. Schaffir, "What are little boys made of?," 516–25.

8. Jan Graffelman and Rolf F. Hoekstra, "A statistical analysis of the effect of warfare on the human secondary sex ratio," *Human Biology* 72 (2000): 433–45.

9. Satoshi Kanazawa, "Violent men have more sons: further evidence for the generalized Trivers-Willard hypothesis," *Journal of Theoretical Biology* 239 (2006): 450–59.

10. Samuel Hough Terry, *Controlling Sex in Generation* (New York: Fowler & Wells, 1885), 75–86.

11. Valerie S. Grant and Sarina Yang, "Achieving women and declining sex ratios," *Human Biology* 75 (2003): 917–27.

12. Marianne E. Bernstein, "A genetic explanation of the wartime increase in secondary sex ratio," *American Journal of Human Genetics* 10 (1958): 68–70.

13. William H. James, "Cycle day of insemination, coital rate, and sex ratio," *Lancet* 297 (1971): 112–14.

14. Robin E. Hilsenrath et al., "Effect of sexual abstinence on the proportion of X-bearing sperm as assessed by multicolor fluorescent in situ hybridization," *Fertility and Sterility* 68 (1997): 510–13.

15. Schaffir, "What are little boys made of?," 516–25.

16. Allen J. Wilcox, Clarice R. Weinberg, and Donna D. Baird, "Timing of sexual intercourse in relation to ovulation," *New England Journal of Medicine* 333 (1995): 1517–21.

17. Ronald H. Gray, "Natural family planning and sex selection: fact or fiction?" *American Journal of Obstetrics & Gynecology* 165 (1991): 1982–84.

18. Sally Langendoen and William Proctor, *The Preconception Gender Diet* (New York: M. Evans and Co., 1982), 55–57.

19. Elizabeth M. Whelan, *Boy or Girl? The Sex Selection Technique That Makes All Others Obsolete* (Indianapolis: Bobbs-Merrill, 1978), 61–62.

20. Landrum B. Shettles and David M. Rorvik, *How to Choose the Sex of Your Baby* (New York: Doubleday, 1989), 109–77.

21. Barbara W. Simcock, "Sons and daughters—a sex preselection study," *Medical Journal of Australia* 142 (1985): 541–42.

22. John T. France et al., "A prospective study of the preselection of the sex of offspring by timing intercourse relative to ovulation," *Fertility and Sterility* 41 (1984): 894–900.

23. Valerie J. Grant and Lawrence W. Chamley, "Can mammalian mothers influence the sex of their offspring periconceptually?" *Reproduction* 140 (2010): 425–33.

24. Jena Pincott, *Do Chocolate Lovers Have Sweeter Babies? The Surprising Science of Pregnancy* (New York: Free Press, 2011), 38–41.

25. Fiona Mathews, Paul J. Johnson, and Andrew Neil, "You are what your mother eats: evidence for maternal preconception diet influencing foetal sex in humans," *Proceedings of the Royal Society B* 275 (2008): 1661–68.

26. Langendoen and Proctor, *The Preconception Gender Diet*, 42–43.

27. Langendoen and Proctor, *The Preconception Gender Diet*, 64–131.

28. Joseph Stolkowski and Jacques Lorrain, "Preconceptional selection of fetal sex," *International Journal of Gynaecology and Obstetrics* 18 (1980): 440–43.

29. Christina Ruegsegger Veit and Raphael Jewelewicz, "Gender preselection: facts and myths," *Fertility and Sterility* 49 (1988): 937–40.

30. Annet M. Noorlander, J. P. M. Geraedts, and J. B. M. Melissen, "Female gender pre-selection by maternal diet in combination with timing of sexual intercourse—a prospective study," *Reproductive Medicine Online* 21 (2010): 794–802.

4. GENDER PREDICTION

1. Carol Dunham, *Mamatoto: A Celebration of Birth* (New York: Penguin Books, 1991), 33–36.

2. Saad Ramzi Ismail, "The relationship between placental location and fetal gender (Ramzi's method)," accessed November 15, 2016, http://www.obgyn.net/articles/relationship-between-placental-location-and-fetal-gender-ramzi%E2%80%99s-method .

3. R. M. Jafari et al., "Fetal gender screening based on placental location by 2-dimensional ultrasonography," *Tehran University Medical Journal* 72 (2014): 323–28.

4. Owsei Temkin, *Soranus' Gynecology* (Baltimore: Johns Hopkins Press, 1956), 44–45.

5. Dunham, *Mamatoto*, 33–36.

6. C. Robert Almli, Robert H. Ball, and Mark E. Wheeler, "Human fetal and neonatal movement patterns: gender differences and fetal-to-neonatal continuity," *Developmental Psychobiology* 38 (2001): 252–73.

7. Shu Shu Costa, *Lotus Seeds and Lucky Stars* (New York: Simon & Schuster, 1998), 67–68.

8. Dunham, *Mamatoto*, 33–36.

9. Deborah F. Perry, Janet DiPietro, and Kathleen Costigan, "Are women carrying 'basketballs' really having boys? Testing pregnancy folklore," *Birth* 26 (1999): 172–77.

10. Kek Khee Loo et al., "Dreams of tigers and flowers: child gender predictions in an urban mainland Chinese sample during pregnancy," *Women's Health* 49 (2009): 50–65.

11. Molly Kay Walker and Garris Keels Conner, "Fetal sex preference of second-trimester gravidas," *Journal of Nurse-Midwifery* 38 (1993): 110–13.

12. Stephen Genuis, Shelagh K. Genuis, and Wei-Ching Chang, "Antenatal fetal heart rate and 'maternal intuition' as predictors of fetal sex," *Journal of Reproductive Medicine* 41 (1996): 447–49.

13. Ronit Haimov-Kochman, Yael Sciaky-Tamir, and Arye Hurwitz, "Reproduction concepts and practices mirrored by modern medicine," *European Journal of Obstetrics & Gynecology and Reproductive Biology* 123 (2005): 3–8.

14. P. Ghalioungui, S. H. Khalil, and A. R. Ammar, "On an ancient Egyptian method of diagnosing pregnancy and determining foetal sex," *Medical History* 7 (1962): 241–46.

15. Robert M. Fowler, "The Drano test," *Journal of the American Medical Association* 248 (1982): 831.

16. Sarah Ostler and Anna Sun, "Fetal sex determination: the predictive value of 3 common myths," *Canadian Medical Association Journal* 161 (1999): 1525–26.

17. Dena Goffman et al., "The accuracy of gender prediction tools," *Obstetrics & Gynecology* 109 Suppl 4 (2007): 42S.

18. Ostler and Sun, "Fetal sex determination," 1525–26.

19. Johan Askling et al., "Sickness in pregnancy and sex of child," *Lancet* 354 (1999): 2053.

20. Melissa A. Schiff, Susan D. Reed, and Janet R. Daling, "The sex ratio of pregnancies complicated by hospitalisation for hyperemesis gravidarum," *British Journal of Obstetrics & Gynaecology* 111 (2004): 27–30.

21. Rulla M. Tamimi et al., "Average energy intake among pregnant women carrying a boy compared with a girl," *BMJ: British Medical Journal* 326 (2003): 1245–46.

22. J. R. Cain, Ursula K. Abbott, and V. L. Rogallo, "Heart rate of the developing chick embryo," *Proceedings of the Society for Experimental Biology and Medicine* 126 (1967): 507–10.

23. A. Charpentier, *Cyclopaedia of Obstetrics and Gynecology*, vol. 1. (New York: William Wood & Co., 1887), 278.

24. L. W. Sontag and T. W. Richards, "Studies in fetal behavior: I. Fetal heart rate as a behavioral indicator," *Monographs of the Society for Research in Child Development* 3 (1938): 1–69.

25. Genuis et al., "Antenatal fetal heart rate," 447–49.

26. Terry J. Dubose et al., "Fetal heart rate is not an indicator of the baby's sex," *Journal of Ultrasound in Medicine* 7 (1988): 237–38.

27. Naohiro Tezuka et al., "Development and sexual difference in embryonic heart rates in pregnancies resulting from in vitro fertilization," *Gynecological and Obstetrical Investigation* 46 (1998): 217–19.

28. Bruce Petrie and Sidney J. Segalowitz, "Use of fetal heart rate, other perinatal and maternal factors as predictors of sex," *Perceptual and Motor Skills* 50 (1980): 871–74.

29. Nicholas W. Dawes et al., "Fetal heart rate patterns in term labor vary with sex, gestational age, epidural anesthesia and fetal weight," *American Journal of Obstetrics & Gynecology* 180 (1999): 181–87.

5. FOOD AVERSIONS AND CRAVINGS

1. Beverley O'Brien and Niles Newton, "Psyche versus soma: historical evolution of beliefs about nausea and vomiting during pregnancy," *Journal of Psychosomatic Obstetrics and Gynecology* 12 (1991): 91–120.

2. Gideon Koren, Svetlana Madjunkova, and Caroline Maltepe, "The protective effects of nausea and vomiting of pregnancy against adverse fetal outcome—a systematic review," *Reproductive Toxicology* 47 (2014): 77–80.

3. Natalia C. Orloff and Julia M. Hormes, "Pickles and ice cream! Food cravings in pregnancy: hypotheses, preliminary evidence, and directions for future research," *Frontiers in Psychology* 5 (2014): 1–15.

4. Jena Pincott, *Do Chocolate Lovers Have Sweeter Babies? The Surprising Science of Pregnancy* (New York: Free Press, 2011), 6.

5. Susan Kruger and Linda Dore Maetzold, "Practices of tradition for pregnancy," *Maternal-Child Nursing Journal* 12 (1983): 135–39.

6. Pincott, *Do Chocolate Lovers Have Sweeter Babies?*, 142–44.

7. O'Brien and Newton, "Psyche versus soma," 91–120.

8. I. Snapper, "Midwifery, past and present," *Bulletin of the New York Academy of Medicine* 39 (1963): 503–32.

9. Kathleen A. Costigan, Heather L. Sipsma, and Janet A. DiPietro, "Pregnancy folklore revisited: the case of heartburn and hair," *Birth* 33 (2006): 311–14.

10. Orloff and Hormes, "Pickles and ice cream," 1–15.

11. Monica H. Green, *The Trotula: An English Translation of the Medieval Compendium of Women's Medicine* (Philadelphia: University of Pennsylvania Press, 2002), 77.

12. Francois Mauriceau, *The Diseases of Women with Child, and in Childbed* (London: John Darby, 1683), 15.

13. Frederick Hollick, *The Marriage Guide, or Natural History of Generation* (New York: TW Strong, 1850), 295.

14. Julius Preuss, *Biblical and Talmudic Medicine* (New York: Sanhedrin Press, 1978), 382.

15. A. J. Hill and D. R. McCance, "Anthropometric and nutritional associations of food cravings in pregnancy," *Pregnancy Hypertension: An International Journal of Women's Cardiovascular Health* 4 (2014): 235.

16. Alexander Woywodt and Akos Kiss, "Geophagia: the history of earth-eating," *Journal of the Royal Society of Medicine* 95 (2002): 143–46.

17. Janet Golden, "The woman who mistook her husband for a steak: the medical legends of morbid 'longings,'" *ACOG Clinical Review* (2000): 12–15.

18. Loudell F. Snow, Shirley M. Johnson, and Harry E. Mayhew, "The behavioral implications of some old wives' tales," *Obstetrics & Gynecology* 51 (1978): 727–32.

19. Sera L. Young, "Pica in pregnancy: new ideas about an old condition," *Annual Review of Nutrition* 30 (2010): 403–22.

6. PRENATAL INFLUENCES

1. Janet L. Sha, *Mothers of Thyme: Customs and Rituals of Infertility and Miscarriage* (Minneapolis: Lida Rose Press, 1990): 77–84.

2. John M. Riddle, *Contraception and Abortion from the Ancient World to the Renaissance* (Cambridge, MA: Harvard University Press, 1994), 9.

3. Owsei Temkin, *Soranus' Gynecology* (Baltimore: Johns Hopkins Press, 1956), 45–49.

4. Francois Mauriceau, *The Diseases of Women with Child and in Childbed*, 2nd ed (Originally published: London: John Darby, 1683; republished in Classics of Medicine Library, Delanco, NJ, 2000), 61–62.

5. Lucille F. Newman, "Folklore of pregnancy: wives' tales in Contra Costa County, California," *Western Folklore* 28 (1969): 112–35.

6. Pye Henry Chavasse, *Advice to a Wife,* 12th ed. (Philadelphia: J.B. Lippincott & Co., 1871), 175–76.

7. Michaell Maia Schlussel et al., "Physical activity during pregnancy and maternal-child health outcomes: a systematic literature review," *Cad Saude Publica* 24 Suppl 4 (2008): S531–44.

8. Mary Latka, Jennie Kline, and Maureen Hatch, "Exercise and spontaneous abortion of known karyotype," *Epidemiology* 10 (1999): 73–75.

9. Laura Fenster et al., "A prospective study of work-related physical exertion and spontaneous abortion," *Epidemiology* 8 (1997): 66–74.

10. Dennis B. McGilvray, "Sexual power and fertility in Sri Lanka: Batticaloa Tamils and Moors," in *Ethnography of Fertility and Birth*, 2nd ed., ed. Carol P. MacCormack (Prospect Heights, IL: Waveland Press, 1994), 15–64.

11. Carol Dunham, *Mamatoto: a Celebration of Birth* (New York: Penguin Books, 1993), 43.

12. Sheila Kitzinger, "The social context of birth: some comparisons between childbirth in Jamaica and Britain," in *Ethnography of Fertility and Birth*, 2nd ed., ed. Carol P. MacCormack (Prospect Heights, IL: Waveland Press, 1994), 171–94.

13. Sarah A. Robertson et al., "Activating T regulatory cells for tolerance in early pregnancy—the contribution of seminal fluid," *Journal of Reproductive Immunology* 83 (2009): 109–16.

14. Jena Pincott, *Do Chocolate Lovers Have Sweeter Babies? The Surprising Science of Pregnancy* (New York: Free Press, 2011), 137–38.

15. Loudell F. Snow, Shirley M. Johnson, and Harry E. Mayhew, "The behavioral implications of some old wives' tales," *Obstetrics & Gynecology* 51 (1978): 727–32.

16. J. H. Pearn and Helen Pavlin, "Maternal impression in a modern Australian community," *Medical Journal of Australia* 2 (1971): 1123–26.

17. Jonathan Schaffir, "Do patients associate adverse pregnancy outcomes with folkloric beliefs?" *Archives of Women's Mental Health* 10 (2007): 301–4.

18. Ambroise Pare, *On Monsters and Marvels*, trans. Janis L. Pallister (Chicago: University of Chicago Press, 1982), 9.

19. L. Lewis Wall, "The strange case of Mary Toft (who was delivered of sixteen rabbits and a tabby cat in 1726)," *Medical Heritage* 3 (1985): 199–212.

20. Philip K. Wilson, "'Out of sight, out of mind?' The Daniel Turner–James Blondel dispute over the power of the maternal imagination," *Annals of Science* 49 (1992): 63–85.

21. William C. Dabney, "Maternal impressions," in *Cyclopaedia of the Diseases of Children*, vol. I., ed. J. M. Keating (Philadelphia: J.B. Lippincott Co., 1889), 191–216.

22. James G. Kiernan, "Maternal impressions," *Journal of the American Medical Association* 33 (1899): 1491.

23. Josef Warkany and Harold Kalter, "Maternal impressions and congenital malformations," *Plastic and Reconstructive Surgery* 30 (1962): 628–37.

24. Sanford Rosenzweig, "Psychological stress in cleft palate etiology," *Journal of Dental Research* 6 Suppl (1966): 1585–593.

25. Dorthe Hansen, Hans C. Lou, and Jorn Olsen, "Serious life events and congenital malformations: a national study with complete follow-up," *Lancet* 356 (2000): 875–80.

26. Suzan L. Carmichael et al., "Maternal stressful life events and risks of birth defects," *Epidemiology* 18 (2007): 356–61.

7. LENGTH OF PREGNANCY

1. Ann Ellis Hanson, "The eight months' child and the etiquette of birth: *obsit omen!*" *Bulletin of the History of Medicine* 61 (1987): 589–602.

2. Rosemary E. Reiss and Avner D. Ash, "The eighth-month fetus: classical sources for a modern superstition," *Obstetrics & Gynecology* 71 (1988): 270–73.

3. Norman M. Ford, *When Did I Begin? Conception of the Human Individual in History, Philosophy and Science* (Cambridge: Cambridge University Press, 1988), 27–28.

4. Julius Preuss, *Biblical and Talmudic Medicine* (New York: Sanhedrin Press, 1978), 389–90.

5. Lars J. Vatten and Rolv Skjaerven, "Offspring sex and pregnancy outcome by length of gestation," *Early Human Development* 76 (2004): 47–54.

6. Gian Carlo di Renzo et al., "Does fetal sex affect pregnancy outcome?" *Gender Medicine* 4 (2007): 19–30.

7. Ingemar Ingemarsson, "Gender aspects of preterm birth," *British Journal of Obstetrics and Gynaecology* 110 (2003): 34–38.

8. Jody L. Zisk et al., "Do premature female infants really do better than their male counterparts?" *American Journal of Perinatology* 28 (2011): 241–46.

9. Thomas F. Baskett and Fritz Naegele, "Naegele's rule: a reappraisal," *British Journal of Obstetrics and Gynaecology* 107 (2000): 1433–35.

10. Per Bergsjo et al., "Duration of human singleton pregnancy—a population-based study," *Acta Obstetricia et Gynecologica Scandinavica* 69 (1990): 197–207.

11. Robert Mittendorf et al., "Predictors of human gestational length," *American Journal of Obstetrics & Gynecology* 168 (1993): 480–84.

12. Allen Downey, "Probably overthinking it: first babies are more likely to be late," accessed October 7, 2016, http://allendowney.blogspot.com/2015/09/first-babies-are-more-likely-to-be-late.html.

13. Spacefem.com, "Due date statistics: a study on the length of pregnancy," accessed November 8, 2016, http://spacefem.com/pregnant/charts/duedate6.php.

8. INDUCING LABOR

1. Zaid Chaudhry, Jane Fischer, and Jonathan Schaffir, "Women's use of nonprescribed methods to induce labor: a brief report," *Birth* 38 (2011): 2–6.

2. George J. Engelmann, "Pregnancy, parturition, and childbed among primitive people," *American Journal of Obstetrics* 14 (1881): 602–18.

3. Howard W. Haggard, *Devils, Drugs and Doctors* (New York: Harper & Bros, 1929), 8–12.

4. Anna Maria Siega-Riz et al., "Frequency of eating during pregnancy and its effect on preterm delivery," *American Journal of Epidemiology* 153 (2001): 647–52.

5. Michael Kaplan, Arthur I. Eidelman, and Yeshaya Aboulafia, "Fasting and the precipitation of labor: the Yom Kippur effect," *Journal of the American Medical Association* 250 (1983): 1317–18.

6. Shu Shu Costa, *Lotus Seeds and Lucky Stars* (New York: Simon & Schuster, 1998), 74–75.

7. Jonathan Schaffir, "Survey of folk beliefs about induction of labor," *Birth* 29 (2002): 47–51.

8. Francois Mauriceau, *The Diseases of Women with Child, and in Childbed* (London: John Darby, 1683), 174.

9. James F. Clapp, "The course of labor after endurance exercise during pregnancy," *American Journal of Obstetrics & Gynecology* 163 (1990): 1799–805.

10. Anne Marie Jukic et al., "A prospective study of the association between vigorous physical activity during pregnancy and length of gestation and birth-weight," *Maternal and Child Health Journal* 16 (2012): 1031–44.

11. Chaudhry et al., "Women's use of nonprescribed methods to induce labor," 2–6.

12. Marit L. Bovbjerg et al., "What started your labor? Responses from mothers in the third Pregnancy, Infection, and Nutrition study," *Journal of Perinatal Education* 23 (2014): 155–64.

13. Henci Goer, "Does walking enhance labor progress?" *Birth* 26 (1999): 127–29.

14. William P. Dewees, *A Treatise on the Diseases of Females*, 4th ed. (Philadelphia: Carey, Lea & Blanchard, 1833), 199.

15. J. Whitridge Williams, *Obstetrics: A Textbook for the Use of Students and Practitioners*, 6th ed. (New York: Appleton & Co., 1930), 457–65.

16. David Garry et al., "Use of castor oil in pregnancies at term," *Alternative Therapies in Health and Medicine* 6 (2000): 77–79.

17. Lorna Davis, "The use of castor oil to stimulate labor in patients with premature rupture of membranes," *Journal of Nurse-Midwifery* 29 (1984): 366–70.

18. Maureen Harris and Maureen Nye, "Self-administration of castor oil," *Modern Midwife* 4 (1994): 29–30.

19. Sonia Hernandez-Diaz et al., "Triggers of spontaneous preterm labor— why today?" *Paediatric and Perinatal Epidemiology* 28 (2014): 79–87.

20. Denise Tiran, "Use of pineapple for induction of labour," *The Practising Midwife* 12 (2009): 33–34.

21. Schaffir, "Survey of folk beliefs," 47–51.

22. Chaudhry et al., "Women's use of nonprescribed methods to induce labor," 2–6.

23. J. I. B. Adinma, "Sexuality in Nigerian pregnant women: perceptions and practice," *Australian and New Zealand Journal of Obstetrics and Gynaecology* 35 (1995): 290–93.

24. Maryam Naim and Erum Bhutto, "Sexuality during pregnancy in Pakistani women," *Journal of the Pakistan Medical Association* 50 (2000): 38–44.

25. Sheila Kitzinger, "The social context of birth: some comparisons between childbirth in Jamaica and Britain," In *Ethnography of Fertility and Birth*, 2nd ed. Carol P. MacCormack (Prospect Heights, IL: Waveland Press, 1994), 171–194.

26. Jonathan Schaffir, "Sexual intercourse at term and onset of labor," *Obstetrics & Gynecology* 107 (2006): 1310–14.

27. Peng Chiong Tan, Choon Ming Yow, and Siti Zawiah Omar, "Effect of coital activity on onset of labor in women scheduled for labor induction: a randomized controlled trial," *Obstetrics & Gynecology* 110 (2007): 820–26; Noorkardiffa Syawalina Omar et al., "Coitus to expedite the onset of labour: a randomized trial," *British Journal of Obstetrics and Gynaecology* 120 (2013): 338–45.

28. Josephine Kavanagh, Anthony J. Kelly, and Jane Thomas, "Breast stimulation for cervical ripening and induction of labour," *Cochrane Database of Systematic Reviews* 2005, Issue 3, Art. No.: CD003392.

29. Maggie Evans, "Postdates pregnancy and complementary therapies," *Complementary Therapies in Clinical Practice* 15 (2009): 220–24.

30. Deborah Hughes, "Birth and the moon," *Modern Midwife* 5 (1995): 28–30.

31. Jonathan Schaffir, "Birth rate and its correlation with the lunar cycle and specific atmospheric conditions," letter to the editor, *American Journal of Obstetrics & Gynecology* 195 (2006): 878.

32. R. Martens, I. W. Kelly, and D. H. Saklofske, "Lunar phase and birthrate: a 50-year critical review," *Psychological Reports* 63 (1998): 923–34.

33. Kenneth L. Noller, Laurence J. Resseguie, and Valerie Voss, "The effect of changes in atmospheric pressure on the occurrence of the spontaneous onset of labor in term pregnancies," *American Journal of Obstetrics & Gynecology* 174 (1996): 1192–99.

34. Susan Morton-Pradhan, R. Curtis Bay, and Dean V. Coonrod, "Birth rate and its correlation with the lunar cycle and specific atmospheric conditions," *American Journal of Obstetrics & Gynecology* 192 (2005): 1970–73.

35. Georgeann H. Polansky, Michael W. Varner, and Tom O'Gorman, "Premature rupture of the membranes and barometric pressure changes," *Journal of Reproductive Medicine* 30 (1985): 189–91.

36. Spyros Milingos et al., "Influence of meteorological factors on premature rupture of fetal membranes," *Lancet* 2 (1978): 435.

9. EASING LABOR

1. M. Erica Couto-Ferreira, "She will give birth easily: therapeutic approaches to childbirth in 1st millennium BCE cuneiform sources," *Dynamis* 32 (2014): 289–315.

2. Rosalind Franklin, *Baby Lore: Superstitions & Old Wives Tales from the World Over Related to Pregnancy, Birth & Babycare* (West Sussex, UK: Diggory Press, 2005), 83–86.

3. Tim Clark, "How to have a baby," *The Old Farmers' Almanac* online, accessed November 11, 2016, www.almanac.com/content/how-have-baby.

4. George J. Engelmann, "Pregnancy, parturition, and childbed among primitive people," *American Journal of Obstetrics* 14 (1881): 828–47.

5. Annemarie Lawrence et al., "Maternal positions and mobility during first stage labour," *Cochrane Database of Systematic Reviews* 2013, Issue 10, Art No: CD003934.

6. Christine L. Roberts, Charles S. Algert, and Emily Olive, "Impact of first-stage ambulation on mode of delivery among women with epidural analgesia," *Australian and New Zealand Journal of Obstetrics and Gynaecology* 44 (2004): 489–94.

7. John M. Riddle, "Artemisia, the 'mother herb,'" in *Goddesses, Elixirs, and Witches: Plants and Sexuality throughout Human History*, ed. John M. Riddle (New York: Palgrave Macmillan, 2010), 79–112.

8. Hugo J. de Boer and Crystle Cotingting, "Medicinal plants for women's healthcare in southeast Asia: a meta-analysis of their traditional use, chemical constituents, and pharmacology," *Journal of Ethnopharmacology* 151 (2014): 747–67.

9. Izharul Hasan et al., "History of ancient Egyptian obstetrics & gynecology: a review," *Journal of Microbiology and Biotechnology Research* 1 (2011): 35–39.

10. Quran 19:24, as translated in *The Noble Qur'an* online, accessed November 1, 2016, www.quran.com.

11. O. Al-Kuran et al., "The effect of late pregnancy consumption of date fruit on labour and delivery," *Journal of Obstetrics and Gynaecology* 31 (2011): 29–31.

12. J. H. Burn and E. R. Withell, "A principle in raspberry leaves which relaxes uterine muscle," *Lancet* 238 (1941): 1–3.

13. Michele Simpson et al., "Raspberry leaf in pregnancy: its safety and efficacy in labor," *Journal of Midwifery & Women's Health* 46 (2001): 51–59.

14. Engelmann, "Pregnancy, parturition and childbed among primitive people," 828–47.

15. Donald Todman, "Childbirth in ancient Rome: from traditional folklore to obstetrics," *Australian and New Zealand Journal of Obstetrics and Gynaecology* 47 (2007): 82–85.

16. Franklin, *Baby Lore*, 83–86.

17. Thomas J. Garite et al., "A randomized controlled trial of the effect of increased intravenous hydration on the course of labor in nulliparous women,"

American Journal of Obstetrics & Gynecology 183 (2000): 1544–48; Feroza Dawood, Therese Dowswell, and Siobhan Quenby, "Intravenous fluids for reducing the duration of labour in low risk nulliparous women," *Cochrane Database of Systematic Reviews* 2013, Issue 6, Art No.: CD007715.

18. A. Kavitha et al., "A randomized controlled trial to study the effect of IV hydration on the duration of labor in nulliparous women," *Archives in Gynecology and Obstetrics* 285 (2012): 343–46.

19. Couto-Ferreira, "She will give birth easily," 289–315.

20. Todman, "Childbirth in ancient Rome," 82–85.

21. American College of Obstetricians and Gynecologists, "Prevention and management of obstetric lacerations at vaginal delivery. Practice Bulletin No. 165," *Obstetrics & Gynecology* 128 (2016): e1–15.

22. Carol Dunham, *Mamatoto: A Celebration of Birth* (New York: Penguin Books, 1991), 89–94.

23. M. Pierce Rucker, "An eighteenth century method of pain relief in obstetrics," *Journal of the History of Medicine* (1950): 101–5.

24. Katherine W. Arendt and Jennifer A. Tessmer-Tuck, "Nonpharmacologic labor analgesia," *Clinics in Perinatology* 40 (2013): 351–71.

25. Caroline A. Smith et al., "Complementary and alternative therapies for pain management in labour," *Cochrane Database of Systematic Reviews* 2006, Issue 4, Art No.: CD003521.

26. Caroline A. Smith et al., "Relaxation techniques for pain management in labour," *Cochrane Database of Systematic Reviews* 2011, Issue 12, Art No.: CD009514.

27. Vincenzo Berghella, Jason K. Baxter, and Suneet P. Chauhan, "Evidence-based labor and delivery management," *American Journal of Obstetrics & Gynecology* 199 (2008): 445–54.

28. I. Snapper, "Midwifery, past and present," *Bulletin of the New York Academy of Medicine* 39 (1963): 503–32.

29. Lucille F. Newman, "Folklore of pregnancy: wives' tales in Contra Costa County, California," *Western Folklore* 28 (1969): 112–35.

30. Engelmann, "Pregnancy, parturition and childbed among primitive people," 828–47.

31. Timothy J. Bungum et al., "Exercise during pregnancy and type of delivery in nulliparae," *Journal of Obstetric, Gynecologic and Neonatal Nursing* 29 (2000): 258–64.

32. Iris Domenjoz, Bengt Kayser, and Michel Boulvain, "Effect of physical activity during pregnancy on mode of delivery," *American Journal of Obstetrics & Gynecology* 211 (2014): 401.e1–11.

10. AFTER BIRTH

1. Sarah J. Buckley, "Placenta rituals and folklore from around the world," *Midwifery Today* 68 (2006): 58–59; E. Croft Long, "The placenta in lore and legend," *Bulletin of the Medical Library Association* 51 (1963): 233–41.

2. Jodi Selander et al., "Human maternal placetophagy: a survey of self-reported motivations and experiences associated with placental consumption," *Ecology of Food and Nutrition* 52 (2013): 93–115.

3. Cynthia W. Coyle et al., "Placentophagy: therapeutic miracle or myth?" *Archives of Women's Mental Health* 18 (2015): 673–80.

4. Stuart B. Blakely, "Superstitions in Obstetrics," *New York State Journal of Medicine* 22 (1922): 349–53.

5. William B. Ober, "Notes on placentophagy," *Bulletin of the New York Academy of Medicine* 55 (1979): 591–99.

6. Michelle Beacock, "Does eating placenta offer postpartum health benefits?" *British Journal of Midwifery* 20 (2012): 464–69.

7. Pranee C. Lundberg and Trieu Thi Ngoc Thu, "Vietnamese women's cultural beliefs and practices related to the postpartum period," *Midwifery* 27 (2011): 731–36.

8. Ushvendra Kaur Choudhry, "Traditional practices of women from India: pregnancy, childbirth, and newborn care," *Journal of Obstetrical, Gynecological, and Neonatal Nursing* 26 (1997): 533–39.

9. Emine Geckil, Turkan Sahin, and Emel Ege, "Traditional postpartum practices of women and infants and the factors influencing such practices in Southeastern Turkey," *Midwifery* 25 (2009): 62–71.

10. Yeoun Soo Kim-Godwin, "Postpartum beliefs and practices among non-Western cultures," *American Journal of Maternal/ Child Nursing* 28 (2003): 74–80.

11. Mary N. Marquez and Consuelo Pacheco, "Midwifery lore in New Mexico," *American Journal of Nursing* 64 (1964): 81–84.

12. Michele R. Forman et al., "The forty-day rest period and infant feeding practices among Negev Bedouin Arab women in Israel," *Medical Anthropology* 12 (1990): 207–16.

13. Natalie Knodel, "Reconsidering an obsolete rite: the churching of women and feminist liturgical theology," *Feminist Theology* 5 (1997): 106–25.

14. A. Charpentier, *Cyclopaedia of Obstetrics and Gynecology*, vol. 1, trans. Egbert H. Grandin (New York: William Wood & Co, 1887), 504.

15. Yan Qun Liu, Marcia Petrini, and Judith A. Maloni, "'Doing the month': postpartum practices in Chinese women," *Nursing and Health Sciences* 17 (2015): 5–14.

16. Yan Qun Liu, Judith A. Maloni, and Marcia Petrini, "Effect of postpartum practices of doing the month on Chinese women's physical and psychological health," *Biological Research for Nursing* 16 (2014): 55–63.

17. Kelly R. Evenson et al., "Summary of international guidelines for physical activity after pregnancy," *Obstetrical and Gynecological Survey* 69 (2014): 407–14.

18. Lucas Minig et al., "Building the evidence base for postoperative and postpartum advice," *Obstetrics & Gynecology* 114 (2009): 892–900.

19. Jane Mutambirwa, "Pregnancy, childbirth, mother and child care among the indigenous people of Zimbabwe," *International Journal of Obstetrics and Gynaecology* 23 (1985): 275–85.

20. Lawrence M. Leeman and Rebecca G. Rogers, "Sex after childbirth: postpartum sexual function," *Obstetrics & Gynecology* 119 (2012): 647–55.

21. A. Cullen Richardson et al., "Decreasing postpartum sexual abstinence time," *American Journal of Obstetrics & Gynecology* 126 (1976): 416–17.

11. BREASTFEEDING

1. Marie Walter, "The folklore of breastfeeding," *Bulletin of the New York Academy of Medicine* 51 (1975): 870–76.

2. Jonathan Schaffir and Cheryl Czapla, "Survey of lactation instructors on folk traditions in breastfeeding," *Breastfeeding Medicine* 7 (2012): 230–33.

3. J. Lewis Smith, *A Treatise on the Diseases of Infancy and Childhood* (Philadelphia: Henry Lea, 1872), 47.

4. Julie A. Mennella and Gary K. Beauchamp, "Beer, breast feeding, and folklore," *Developmental Psychobiology* 26 (1993): 459–66.

5. Seham Ragheb and Eleanor W. Smith, "Beliefs and customs regarding breast feeding among Egyptian women in Alexandria," *International Journal of Nursing Studies* 16 (1979): 73–83.

6. Julius Preuss, *Biblical and Talmudic Medicine* (New York: Sanhedrin Press, 1978), 409.

7. Julie A. Mennella, "Alcohol's effect on lactation," *Alcohol Research & Health* 25 (2001): 230–34.

8. Julie A. Mennella and Gary K. Beauchamp, "Maternal diet alters the sensory qualities of human milk and the behavior of the nursling," *Pediatrics* 88 (1991): 737–44.

9. Elmer R. Grossman, "Beer, breastfeeding, and the wisdom of old wives," *Journal of the American Medical Association* 259 (1988): 1016.

10. Berthold Koletzko and Frauke Lehner, "Beer and breastfeeding," *Advances in Experimental Medicine and Biology* 478 (2000): 23–28.

11. Monica H. Green, *The Trotula: an English Translation of the Medieval Compendium of Women's Medicine* (Philadelphia: University of Pennsylvania Press, 2002), 84–85.

12. Smith. *A Treatise on the Diseases of Infancy and Childhood*, 47.

13. Schaffir and Czapla, "Survey of lactation instructors on folk traditions," 230–33.

14. Francesco Di Pierro et al., "Clinical efficacy, safety and tolerability of BIO-C (micronized silymarin) as a galactogogue," *Acta Biomedica* 79 (2008): 205–10.

15. Marina Heilmeyer, *Ancient Herbs* (Los Angeles: Getty Publications, 2007), 50.

16. Georgios A. Petropoulos, *Fenugreek: The Genus Trigonella* (Boca Raton: CRC Press, 2003), 1–2.

17. Antonio Alberto Zuppa et al., "Safety and efficacy of galactogogues: substances that induce, maintain and increase breast milk production," *Journal of Pharmacy and Pharmaceutical Sciences* 13 (2010): 162–74.

18. William P. Dewees, *A Treatise on the Diseases of Females*, 4th ed. (Philadelphia: Carey & Lea, 1833), 503–4.

19. Beatrice Fontanel and Claire d'Harcourt, *Babies: History, Art and Folklore* (New York: Harry Abrams, 1997), 112.

20. Francois Mauriceau, *The Diseases of Women with Child, and in Childbed* (London: John Darby, 1683), 341.

21. Smriti Arora, Manju Vatsa, and Vatsla Dadhwal, "A comparison of cabbage leaves vs hot and cold compresses in the treatment of breast engorgement, *Indian Journal of Community Medicine* 33 (2008): 160–62.

22. V. Cheryl Nikodem et al., "Do cabbage leaves prevent breast engorgement? A randomized, controlled study," *Birth* 20 (1993): 61–64.

23. Kathryn L. Roberts, Maureen Reiter, and Diane Schuster, "A comparison of chilled and room temperature cabbage leaves in treating breast engorgement," *Journal of Human Lactation* 11 (1995): 191–94.

24. Kathryn L. Roberts, Maureen Reiter, and Diane Schuster, "Effects of cabbage leaf extract on breast engorgement," *Journal of Human Lactation* 14 (1998): 231–36.

25. Lindeka Mangesi and Therese Dowswell, "Treatments for breast engorgement during lactation," *Cochrane Database of Systematic Reviews* 2010, Issue 9, Art No.: CD006946.

26. Noelie A. Lavergne, "Does application of tea bags to sore nipples while breastfeeding provide effective relief?" *Journal of Obstetric, Gynecologic and Neonatal Nursing* 26 (1997): 53–58.

27. Kristine Morland-Schultz and Pamela D. Hill, "Prevention of and therapies for nipple pain: a systemic review," *Journal of Obstetric, Gynecologic and Neonatal Nursing* 34 (2005): 428–37.

28. Fontanel and d'Harcourt, *Babies*, 95.

29. Owsei Temkin, *Soranus' Gynecology* (Baltimore: Johns Hopkins Press, 1956), 99.

30. Green, *The Trotula*, 84–85.

31. Helene Hausner et al., "Differential transfer of dietary flavour compounds into human breast milk," *Physiology & Behavior* 95 (2008): 118–24.

32. Katherine D. Lust, Judith E. Brown, and William Thomas, "Maternal intake of cruciferous vegetables and other foods and colic symptoms in exclusively breast-fed infants," *Journal of the American Dietary Association* 96 (1996): 47–48.

BIBLIOGRAPHY

Adinma, J. I. B. "Sexuality in Nigerian pregnant women: perceptions and practice." *Australian and New Zealand Journal of Obstetrics & Gynaecology* 35 (1995): 290–93.

Al-Kuran, O., L. Al-Mehaisen, H. Bawadi, S. Beitawi, and Z. Amarin. "The effect of late pregnancy consumption of date fruit on labour and delivery." *Journal of Obstetrics & Gynaecology* 31 (2011): 29–31.

Almli, C. Robert, Robert H. Ball, and Mark E. Wheeler. "Human fetal and neonatal movement patterns: gender differences and fetal-to-neonatal continuity." *Developmental Psychobiology* 38 (2001): 252–73.

American College of Obstetricians and Gynecologists. "Prevention and management of obstetric lacerations at vaginal delivery. Practice Bulletin No. 165." *Obstetrics & Gynecology* 128 (2016): e1–15.

Arendt, Katherine W., and Jennifer A. Tessmer-Tuck. "Nonpharmacologic labor analgesia." *Clinics in Perinatology* 40 (2013): 351–71.

Arora, Smriti, Manju Vatsa, and Vatsla Dadhwal. "A comparison of cabbage leaves vs hot and cold compresses in the treatment of breast engorgement." *Indian Journal of Community Medicine* 33 (2008): 160–62.

Askling, Johan, Gunnar Erlandsson, Magnus Kaijser, Olof Akre, and Anders Ekbom. "Sickness in pregnancy and sex of child." *Lancet* 354 (1999): 2053.

Baskett, Thomas F., and Fritz Naegele. "Naegele's rule: a reappraisal." *British Journal of Obstetrics & Gynaecology* 107 (2000): 1433–35.

Beacock, Michelle. "Does eating placenta offer postpartum health benefits?" *British Journal of Midwifery* 20 (2012): 464–69.

Bennington, Linda K. "Can complementary/alternative medicine be used to treat infertility?" *American Journal of Maternal/Child Nursing* 35 (2010): 140–47.

Berghella, Vincenzo, Jason K. Baxter, and Suneet P. Chauhan. "Evidence-based labor and delivery management." *American Journal of Obstetrics & Gynecology* 199 (2008): 445–54.

Bergsjo, Per, Daniel W. Denman, Howard J. Hoffman, and Olav Meirik. "Duration of human singleton pregnancy—a population-based study." *Acta Obstetricia et Gynecologica Scandinavica* 69 (1990): 197–207.

Bernstein, Marianne E. "A genetic explanation of the wartime increase in secondary sex ratio." *American Journal of Human Genetics* 10 (1958): 68–70.

Blakely, Stuart B. "Superstitions in Obstetrics." *New York State Journal of Medicine* 22 (1922): 349–53.

Boivin, Jacky, Janet E. Takefman, William Brender, and Togas Tulandi. "The effects of female sexual response in coitus on early reproductive processes." *Journal of Behavioral Medicine* 15 (1992): 509–18.

Bovbjerg, Marit L., Kelly R. Evenson, Chyrise Bradley, and John M. Thorp, Jr. "What started your labor? Responses from mothers in the third Pregnancy, Infection, and Nutrition study." *Journal of Perinatal Education* 23 (2014): 155–64.

Buckley, Sarah J. "Placenta rituals and folklore from around the world." *Midwifery Today* 68 (2006): 58–59.

Bungum, Timothy J., Dian L. Peaslee, Allen W. Jackson, and Miguel A. Perez. "Exercise during pregnancy and type of delivery in nulliparae." *Journal of Obstetric, Gynecologic and Neonatal Nursing* 29 (2000): 258–64.

Burn, J. H., and E. R. Withell. "A principle in raspberry leaves which relaxes uterine muscle." *Lancet* 238 (1941): 1–3.

Cain, J. R., Ursula K. Abbott, and V. L. Rogallo. "Heart rate of the developing chick embryo." *Proceedings of the Society for Experimental Biology and Medicine* 126 (1967): 507–10.

Carmichael, Suzan L., Gary M. Shaw, Wei Yang, Barbara Abrams, and Edward J. Lammer. "Maternal stressful life events and risks of birth defects." *Epidemiology* 18 (2007): 356–61.

Cha, Kwang Y., Daniel P. Wirth, and Rogerio A. Lobo. "Does prayer influence the success of in vitro fertilization-embryo transfer?" *Journal of Reproductive Medicine* 46 (2001): 781–87.

Charpentier, A. *Cyclopaedia of Obstetrics and Gynecology*, vol. 1. Translated by Egbert H. Grandin. New York: William Wood & Co., 1887.

Chaudhry, Zaid, Jane Fischer, and Jonathan Schaffir. "Women's use of nonprescribed methods to induce labor: a brief report." *Birth* 38 (2011): 2–6.

Chavarro, Jorge E., Janet W. Rich-Edwards, Bernard A. Rosner, and Walter C. Willett. "Diet and lifestyle in the prevention of ovulatory disorder infertility." *Obstetrics & Gynecology* 110 (2007): 1050–58.

———. "Use of multivitamins, intake of B vitamins, and risk of ovulatory infertility." *Fertility and Sterility* 89 (2008): 668–76.

Chavasse, Pye Henry. *Advice to a Wife*, 12th ed. Philadelphia: J.B. Lippincott & Co., 1871.

Choudhry, Ushvenda Kaur. "Traditional practices of women from India: pregnancy, childbirth, and newborn care," *Journal of Obstetrical, Gynecological, and Neonatal Nursing* 26 (1997): 533–39.

Clapp, James F. "The course of labor after endurance exercise during pregnancy." *American Journal of Obstetrics & Gynecology* 163 (1990): 1799–805.

Clark, Tim. "How to have a baby." *The Old Farmers' Almanac* online. Accessed November 11, 2016.www.almanac.com/content/how-have-baby.

Costa, Shu Shu. *Lotus Seeds and Lucky Stars*. New York: Simon & Schuster, 1998.

Costigan, Kathleen A., Heather L. Sipsma, and Janet A. DiPietro. "Pregnancy folklore revisited: the case of heartburn and hair." *Birth* 33 (2006): 311–14.

Couto-Ferreira, M. Erica. "She will give birth easily: therapeutic approaches to childbirth in 1st millennium BCE cuneiform sources." *Dynamis* 32 (2014): 289–315.

Coyle, Cynthia W., Kathryn E. Hulse, Katherine L. Wisner, Kara E. Driscoll, and Crystal T. Clark. "Placentophagy: therapeutic miracle or myth?" *Archives of Women's Mental Health* 18 (2015): 673–80.

Culpeper, Nicholas. *A Directory for Midwives: Or, A Guide to Women in Their Conception, Bearing, and Suckling Their Children*. London: T. Norris, 1724.

Dabney, William C. "Maternal impressions." In *Cyclopaedia of the Diseases of Children*, vol. I, edited by J. M. Keating. Philadelphia: J.B. Lippincott Co., 1889.

Daniele, Claudia, Joanna Thompson Coon, Max H. Pittler, and Edzard Ernst. "Vitex agnus castus: a systematic review of adverse events." *Drug Safety* 28 (2005): 319–32.

Davis, Lorna. "The use of castor oil to stimulate labor in patients with premature rupture of membranes." *Journal of Nurse-Midwifery* 29 (1984): 366–70.

Dawes, Nicholas W., Geoffrey S. Dawes, Mary Moulden, and Christopher W. G. Redman. "Fetal heart rate patterns in term labor vary with sex, gestational age, epidural anesthesia and fetal weight." *American Journal of Obstetrics & Gynecology* 180 (1999): 181–87.

Dawood, Feroza, Therese Dowswell, and Siobhan Quenby. "Intravenous fluids for reducing the duration of labour in low risk nulliparous women." *Cochrane Database of Systematic Reviews* 2013, Issue 6, Art No.: CD007715.

De Boer, Hugo J., and Crystle Cotingting. "Medicinal plants for women's healthcare in southeast Asia: a meta-analysis of their traditional use, chemical constituents, and pharmacology." *Journal of Ethnopharmacology* 151 (2014): 747–67.

Dewees, William P. *A Treatise on the Diseases of Females*, 4th ed. Philadelphia: Carey, Lea & Blanchard, 1833.

Di Pierro, Francesco, Alberto Callegari, Domenico Carotenuto, and Marco Mollo Tapia. "Clinical efficacy, safety and tolerability of BIO-C (micronized silymarin) as a galactogogue." *Acta Biomedica* 79 (2008): 205–10.

Di Renzo, Gian Carlo, Alessia Rosati, Roberta Donati Sarti, Laura Cruciani, and Antonio Massimo Cutuli. "Does fetal sex affect pregnancy outcome?" *Gender Medicine* 4 (2007): 19–30.

Domenjoz, Iris, Bengt Kayser, and Michel Boulvain. "Effect of physical activity during pregnancy on mode of delivery." *American Journal of Obstetrics & Gynecology* 211 (2014): 401.e1–11.

Downey, Allen. "Probably overthinking it: first babies are more likely to be late." Accessed October 7, 2016.http://allendowney.blogspot.com/2015/09/first-babies-are-more-likely-to-be-late.html.

Dubose, Terry J., Denise Dickey, Chris M. Butscher, Linda Porter, Larry W. Hill, and E. K. Poole. "Fetal heart rate is not an indicator of the baby's sex." *Journal of Ultrasound in Medicine* 7 (1988): 237–38.

Dunham, Carol. *Mamatoto: A Celebration of Birth*. New York: Penguin Books, 1991.

Edirne, Tamer, Secil Gunher Arica, Sebahat Gucuk, Recep Yildizhan, Ali Kolusari, Ertan Adali, and Muhammet Can. "Use of complementary and alternative medicines by a sample of Turkish women for infertility enhancement: a descriptive study." *BMC Complementary and Alternative Medicine* 10 (2010): 11–17.

Engelmann, George J. "Pregnancy, parturition, and childbed among primitive people." *American Journal of Obstetrics* 14 (1881): 602–18, 828–47.

Evans, Maggie. "Postdates pregnancy and complementary therapies." *Complementary Therapies in Clinical Practice* 15 (2009): 220–24.

Evenson, Kelly R., Michelle F. Mottola, Katrine M. Owe, Emily K. Rousham, and Wendy J. Brown. "Summary of international guidelines for physical activity after pregnancy." *Obstetrical and Gynecological Survey* 69 (2014): 407–14.

Fenster, Laura, Alan E. Hubbard, Gayle C. Windham, Kirsten O. Waller, and Shanna H. Swan. "A prospective study of work-related physical exertion and spontaneous abortion." *Epidemiology* 8 (1997): 66–74.

Flamm, Bruce L. "Prayer and the success of IVF." *Journal of Reproductive Medicine* 50 (2005): 71.

Fontanel, Beatrice, and Claire d'Harcourt. *Babies: History, Art and Folklore*. New York: Harry Abrams, 1997.

Ford, Norman M. *When Did I Begin? Conception of the Human Individual in History, Philosophy and Science*. Cambridge: Cambridge University Press, 1988.

Forman, Michele R., Gillian L. Hundt, D. Towne, B. Graubard, Barbara Sullivan, Heinz W. Berendes, Batia Sarov, and Lechaim Naggan. "The forty-day rest period and infant feeding practices among Negev Bedouin Arab women in Israel." *Medical Anthropology* 12 (1990): 207–16.

Fowler, Robert M. "The Drano test." *Journal of the American Medical Association* 248 (1982): 831.

France, John T., Frederick M. Graham, Leonie Gosling, and Philip I. Hair. "A prospective study of the preselection of the sex of offspring by timing intercourse relative to ovulation." *Fertility and Sterility* 41 (1984): 894–900.

Franklin, Rosalind. *Baby Lore: Superstitions & Old Wives Tales from the World Over*. Sussex, UK: Diggory Press, 2005.

Garite, Thomas J., Jonathan Weeks, Kimberly Peters-Phair, Carol Pattillo, and Wendy R. Brewster. "A randomized controlled trial of the effect of increased intravenous hydration on the course of labor in nulliparous women." *American Journal of Obstetrics & Gynecology* 183 (2000): 1544–48.

Garry, David, Reinaldo Figueroa, Jacques Guillaume, and Valerie Cucco. "Use of castor oil in pregnancies at term." *Alternative Therapies in Health and Medicine* 6 (2000): 77–79.

Geckil, Emine, Turkan Sahin, and Emel Ege. "Traditional postpartum practices of women and infants and the factors influencing such practices in Southeastern Turkey." *Midwifery* 25 (2009): 62–71.

Genuis, Stephen, Shelagh K. Genuis, and Wei-Ching Chang. "Antenatal fetal heart rate and 'maternal intuition' as predictors of fetal sex." *Journal of Reproductive Medicine* 41 (1996): 447–49.

Ghalioungui, P., S. H. Khalil, and A. R. Ammar. "On an ancient Egyptian method of diagnosing pregnancy and determining foetal sex." *Medical History* 7 (1962): 241–46.

Goer, Henci. "Does walking enhance labor progress?" *Birth* 26 (1999): 127–29.

Goffman, Dena, Temuri Budagov, Gil Atzmon, Brian Wagner, and Francine Einstein. "The accuracy of gender prediction tools." *Obstetrics & Gynecology* 109 (2007): 42S.

Golden, Janet. "The woman who mistook her husband for a steak: the medical legends of morbid "longings." *ACOG Clinical Review* (2000): 12–15.

Graffelman, Jan, and Rolf F. Hoekstra. "A statistical analysis of the effect of warfare on the human secondary sex ratio." *Human Biology* 72 (2000): 433–45.

Grant, Valerie J., and Lawrence W. Chamley. "Can mammalian mothers influence the sex of their offspring periconceptually?" *Reproduction* 140 (2010): 425–33.

Grant, Valerie J., and Sarina Yang. "Achieving women and declining sex ratios." *Human Biology* 75 (2003): 917–27.

Gray, Ronald H. "Natural family planning and sex selection: fact or fiction?" *American Journal of Obstetrics & Gynecology* 165 (1991): 1982–84.

Green, Monica H. *The Trotula: an English Translation of the Medieval Compendium of Women's Medicine*. Philadelphia: University of Pennsylvania Press, 2002.

Grossman, Elmer R. "Beer, breastfeeding, and the wisdom of old wives." *Journal of the American Medical Association* 259 (1988): 1016.

Haggard, Howard W. *Devils, Drugs and Doctors*. New York: Harper & Bros, 1929.

Haimov-Kochman, Ronit, Yael Sciaky-Tamir, and Arye Hurwitz. "Reproduction concepts and practices mirrored by modern medicine." *European Journal of Obstetrics & Gynecology and Reproductive Biology* 123 (2005): 3–8.

Hansen, Dorthe, Hans C. Lou, and Jorn Olsen. "Serious life events and congenital malformations: a national study with complete follow-up." *Lancet* 356 (2000): 875–80.

Hanson, Ann E. "The eight months' child and the etiquette of birth: *obsit omen!*" *Bulletin of the History of Medicine* 61 (1987): 589–602.

Harris, Maureen, and Maureen Nye. "Self-administration of castor oil." *Modern Midwife* 4 (1994): 29–30.

Hasan, Izharul, Mohd Zulkifle, A. H. Ansari, A. M. K. Sherwani, and Mohd Shakir. "History of ancient Egyptian obstetrics and gynecology: a review." *Journal of Microbiology and Biotechnology Research* 1 (2011): 35–39.

Hausner, Helene, Wender L. Bredie, Christian Molgaard, Mikael A. Petersen, and Per Moller. "Differential transfer of dietary flavour compounds into human breast milk." *Physiology & Behavior* 95 (2008): 118–24.

Heilmeyer, Marina. *Ancient Herbs*. Los Angeles: Getty Publications, 2007.

Hernandez-Diaz, Sonia, Caroline E. Boeke, Anna Thornton Romans, Brett Young, Andrea V. Margulis, Thomas F. McElrath, Jeffrey L. Ecker, and Brian T. Bateman. "Triggers of spontaneous preterm labor—why today?" *Paediatric and Perinatal Epidemiology* 28 (2014): 79–87.

Hill, A. J., and D. R. McCance. "Anthropometric and nutritional associations of food cravings in pregnancy." *Pregnancy Hypertension: An International Journal of Women's Cardiovascular Health* 4 (2014): 235.

Hilsenrath, Robin E., John E. Buster, Monte Swarup, Sandra A. Carson, and Farideh Z. Bischoff. "Effect of sexual abstinence on the proportion of X-bearing sperm as assessed by multicolor fluorescent in situ hybridization." *Fertility and Sterility* 68 (1997): 510–13.

Hollick, Frederick. *The Marriage Guide, or Natural History of Generation.* New York: TW Strong, 1850.

Hughes, Deborah. "Birth and the moon." *Modern Midwife* 5 (1995): 28–30.

Ingemarsson, Ingemar. "Gender aspects of preterm birth." *British Journal of Obstetrics & Gynaecology* 110 (2003): 34–38.

Jafari, R. M., M. Barati, S. Bagheri, and Z. Shajirat. "Fetal gender screening based on placental location by 2-dimensional ultrasonography." *Tehran University Medical Journal* 72 (2014): 323–28.

James, William H. "Cycle day of insemination, coital rate, and sex ratio." *Lancet* 297 (1971): 112–14.

Jasienska, Grazyna, Anna Ziomkiewicz, Peter T. Ellison, Susan F. Lipson and Inger Thune. "Large breasts and narrow waists indicate high reproductive potential in women," *Proceedings of the Royal Society of London B* 271 (2004): 1213–17.

Jozsa, Laszlo G. "Obesity in the Paleolithic era." *Hormones* 10 (2011): 241–44.

Jukic, Anne Marie, Kelly R. Evenson, Julie L. Daniels, Amy H. Herring, Allen J. Wilcox, and Katherine E. Hartmann. "A prospective study of the association between vigorous physical activity during pregnancy and length of gestation and birthweight." *Maternal and Child Health Journal* 16 (2012): 1031–44.

Kanazawa, Satoshi. "Violent men have more sons: further evidence for the generalized Trivers-Willard hypothesis." *Journal of Theoretical Biology* 239 (2006): 450–59.

Kaplan, Michael, Arthur I. Eidelman, and Yeshaya Aboulafia. "Fasting and the precipitation of labor: the Yom Kippur effect." *Journal of the American Medical Association* 250 (1983): 1317–18.

Kavanagh, Josephine, Anthony J. Kelly, and Jane Thomas. "Breast stimulation for cervical ripening and induction of labour." *Cochrane Database of Systematic Reviews* 2005, Issue 3, Art No.: CD003392.

Kavitha, A., K. P. Chacko, Elsy Thomas, Swati Rathore, Solomon Christopher, Bivas Biswas, and Jiji Elizabeth Mathews. "A randomized controlled trial to study the effect of IV hydration on the duration of labor in nulliparous women." *Archives in Gynecology and Obstetrics* 285 (2012): 343–46.

Kiernan, James G. "Maternal impressions." *Journal of the American Medical Association* 33 (1899): 1491.

Kim-Godwin, Yeoun Soo. "Postpartum beliefs and practices among non-Western cultures." *American Journal of Maternal/ Child Nursing* 28 (2003): 74–80.

King, Helen. "Food as a symbol in classical Greece." *History Today* 36 (1986): 1–5.

Kitzinger, Sheila. "The social context of birth: some comparisons between childbirth in Jamaica and Britain." In *Ethnography of Fertility and Birth*, 2nd ed., edited by Carol P. MacCormack, 171–94. Prospect Heights, IL: Waveland Press, 1994.

Knodel, Natalie. "Reconsidering an obsolete rite: the churching of women and feminist liturgical theology." *Feminist Theology* 5 (1997): 106–25.

Koletzko, Berthold, and Frauke Lehner. "Beer and breastfeeding." *Advances in Experimental Medicine and Biology* 478 (2000): 23–28.

Koren, Gideon, Svetlana Madjunkova, and Caroline Maltepe. "The protective effects of nausea and vomiting of pregnancy against adverse fetal outcome—a systematic review." *Reproductive Toxicology* 47 (2014): 77–80.

Kruger, Susan, and Linda Dore Maetzold, "Practices of tradition for pregnancy," *Maternal-Child Nursing Journal* 12 (1983): 135–39.

Langendoen, Sally, and William Proctor. *The Preconception Gender Diet.* New York: M. Evans and Co., 1982.

Latka, Mary, Jennie Kline, and Maureen Hatch. "Exercise and spontaneous abortion of known karyotype." *Epidemiology* 10 (1999): 73–75.

Lavergne, Noelie A. "Does application of tea bags to sore nipples while breastfeeding provide effective relief?" *Journal of Obstetric, Gynecologic and Neonatal Nursing* 26 (1997): 53–58.

Lawrence, Annemarie, et al. "Maternal positions and mobility during first stage labour." *Cochrane Database of Systematic Reviews* 2013, Issue 10, Art No.: CD003934.

Leeman, Lawrence M., and Rebecca G. Rogers. "Sex after childbirth: postpartum sexual function." *Obstetrics & Gynecology* 119 (2012): 647–55.

Levin, Roy J. "The physiology of sexual arousal in the human female: a recreational and procreational synthesis." *Archives of Sexual Behavior* 31 (2002): 405–11.

Liu, Yan Qun, Marcia Petrini, and Judith A. Maloni. "'Doing the month': postpartum practices in Chinese women." *Nursing and Health Sciences* 17 (2015): 5–14.

———. "Effect of postpartum practices of doing the month on Chinese women's physical and psychological health." *Biological Research for Nursing* 16 (2014): 55–63.

Long, E. Croft. "The placenta in lore and legend." *Bulletin of the Medical Library Association* 51 (1963): 233–41.

Loo, Kek Khee, Xiying Luo, Hong Su, Angela Presson, and Yan Li. "Dreams of tigers and flowers: child gender predictions in an urban mainland Chinese sample during pregnancy." *Women's Health* 49 (2009): 50–65.

Lundberg, Pranee C., and Trieu Thi Ngoc Thu. "Vietnamese women's cultural beliefs and practices related to the postpartum period." *Midwifery* 27 (2011): 731–36.

Lust, Katherine D., Judith E. Brown, and William Thomas. "Maternal intake of cruciferous vegetables and other foods and colic symptoms in exclusively breast-fed infants." *Journal of the American Dietary Association* 96 (1996): 47–48.

MacCormack, Carol P., ed. *Ethnography of Fertility and Birth*, 2nd ed. Prospect Heights, IL: Waveland Press, 1994.

Mangesi, Lindeka, and Therese Dowswell. "Treatments for breast engorgement during lactation." *Cochrane Database of Systematic Reviews* 2010, Issue 9, Art No.: CD006946.

Marquez, Mary N., and Consuelo Pacheco. "Midwifery lore in New Mexico." *American Journal of Nursing* 64 (1964): 81–84.

Martens, R., I. W. Kelly, and D. H. Saklofske. "Lunar phase and birthrate: a 50-year critical review." *Psychological Reports* 63 (1998): 923–34.

Mathews, Fiona, Paul J. Johnson, and Andrew Neil. "You are what your mother eats: evidence for maternal preconception diet influencing foetal sex in humans." *Proceedings of the Royal Society B* 275 (2008): 1661–68.

Matthiesen, S. M., Y. Frederiksen, H. J. Ingerslev, and R. Zachariae. "Stress, distress and outcome of assisted reproductive technology (ART): a meta-analysis." *Human Reproduction* 26 (2011): 2763–76.

Mauriceau, Francois. *The Diseases of Women with Child, and in Child-bed.* London: John Darby, 1683.

May, Margaret T. *Galen: On the Usefulness of the Parts of the Body.* New York: Cornell University Press, 1968.

McGilvray, Dennis B. "Sexual power and fertility in Sri Lanka: Batticaloa Tamils and Moors." In *Ethnography of Fertility and Birth*, 2nd ed., edited by Carol P. MacCormack, 15–64. Prospect Heights, IL: Waveland Press, 1994.

Mennella, Julie A. "Alcohol's effect on lactation." *Alcohol Research & Health* 25 (2001): 230–34.

Mennella, Julie A., and Gary K. Beauchamp. "Beer, breast feeding, and folklore." *Developmental Psychobiology* 26 (1993): 459–66.

———. "Maternal diet alters the sensory qualities of human milk and the behavior of the nursling." *Pediatrics* 88 (1991): 737–44.

Milingos, Spyros, I. Messinis, D. Diakomanolis, D. Aravantinos, and D. Kaskarelis. "Influence of meteorological factors on premature rupture of fetal membranes." *Lancet* 312 (1978): 435.

Minig, Lucas, Edward L. Trimble, Carlos Sarsotti, Mario M. Sebastiani, and Catherine Y. Spong. "Building the evidence base for postoperative and postpartum advice." *Obstetrics & Gynecology* 114 (2009): 892–900.

Mittendorf, Robert, Michelle A. Williams, Catherine S. Berkey, Ellice Lieberman, and Richard R. Monson. "Predictors of human gestational length." *American Journal of Obstetrics & Gynecology* 168 (1993): 480–84.

Morland-Schultz, Kristine, and Pamela D. Hill. "Prevention of and therapies for nipple pain: a systemic review." *Journal of Obstetric, Gynecologic and Neonatal Nursing* 34 (2005): 428–37.

Morton-Pradhan, Susan, R. Curtis Bay, and Dean V. Coonrod. "Birth rate and its correlation with the lunar cycle and specific atmospheric conditions." *American Journal of Obstetrics & Gynecology* 192 (2005): 1970–73.

Mutambirwa, Jane. "Pregnancy, childbirth, mother and child care among the indigenous people of Zimbabwe." *International Journal of Obstetrics & Gynaecology* 23 (1985): 275–85.

Naim, Maryam, and Erum Bhutto. "Sexuality during pregnancy in Pakistani women." *Journal of the Pakistan Medical Association* 50 (2000): 38–44.

Newman, Lucille F. "Folklore of pregnancy: wives' tales in Contra Costa County, California." *Western Folklore* 28 (1969): 112–35.

Ng, Ernest Hung Yu, Wing Sze So, Jing Gao, Yu Yeuk Wong, and Pak Chung Ho. "The role of acupuncture in the management of subfertility." *Fertility and Sterility* 90 (2008): 1–13.

Nikodem, V. Cheryl, Donna Danziger, Nicky Gebka, A. Metin Gulmezoglu, and G. Justus Hofmeyr. "Do cabbage leaves prevent breast engorgement? A randomized, controlled study." *Birth* 20 (1993): 61–64.

Noller, Kenneth L., Laurence J. Resseguie, and Valerie Voss. "The effect of changes in atmospheric pressure on the occurrence of the spontaneous onset of labor in term pregnancies." *American Journal of Obstetrics & Gynecology* 174 (1996): 1192–99.

Noorlander, Annet M., J. P. M. Geraedts, and J. B. M. Melissen. "Female gender preselection by maternal diet in combination with timing of sexual intercourse—a prospective study." *Reproductive Medicine Online* 21 (2010): 794–802.

Ober, William B. "Notes on placentophagy." *Bulletin of the New York Academy of Medicine* 55 (1979): 591–99.

O'Brien, Beverley, and Niles Newton. "Psyche versus soma: historical evolution of beliefs about nausea and vomiting during pregnancy." *Journal of Psychosomatic Obstetrics and Gynecology* 12 (1991): 91–120.

Olderied, Nan B., Hallgeir Rui, and Kenneth Purvis. "Life styles of men in barren couples and their relationship to sperm quality." *International Journal of Fertility* 37 (1992): 343–49.

Omar, Noorkardiffa Syawalina, Peng Chiong Tan, Nada Sabir, Ezra Sophia Yusop, and Siti Zawiah Omar. "Coitus to expedite the onset of labour: a randomized trial." *British Journal of Obstetrics & Gynaecology* 120 (2013): 338–45.

Orloff, Natalia C., and Julia M. Hormes. "Pickles and ice cream! Food cravings in pregnancy: hypotheses, preliminary evidence, and directions for future research." *Frontiers in Psychology* 5 (2014): 1–15.

Ostler, Sarah, and Anna Sun. "Fetal sex determination: the predictive value of 3 common myths." *Canadian Medical Association Journal* 161 (1999): 1525–26.

Page, T. E. "Regimen I, 27." In *Hippocrates*, vol. 4, translated by W. H. S. Jones. New York: Putnam, 1931.

Pare, Ambroise. *On Monsters and Marvels*. Translated by Janis L. Pallister. Chicago: University of Chicago Press, 1982.

Pearn, J. H., and Helen Pavlin, "Maternal impression in a modern Australian community," *Medical Journal of Australia* 2 (1971): 1123–26.

Pei, Kaiyan, Y. Xu, and Mengchun Jia. "Effect of successive ejaculation on semen analysis parameters in normal men." *Zhonghua Nan Ke Xue* 10 (2004): 667–70.

Perry, Deborah F., Janet DiPietro, and Kathleen Costigan. "Are women carrying 'basketballs' really having boys? Testing pregnancy folklore." *Birth* 26 (1999): 172–77.

Petrie, Bruce, and Sidney J. Segalowitz. "Use of fetal heart rate, other perinatal and maternal factors as predictors of sex." *Perceptual and Motor Skills* 50 (1980): 871–74.

Petropoulos, Georgios A. *Fenugreek: the Genus Trigonella*. Boca Raton: CRC Press, 2003.

Pincott, Jena. *Do Chocolate Lovers Have Sweeter Babies? The Surprising Science of Pregnancy*. New York: Free Press, 2011.

Polansky, Georgeann H., Michael W. Varner, Tom O'Gorman. "Premature rupture of the membranes and barometric pressure changes." *Journal of Reproductive Medicine* 30 (1985): 189–91.

Preuss, Julius. *Biblical and Talmudic Medicine*. New York: Sanhedrin Press, 1978.

Quran 19:24, as translated in *The Noble Qur'an* online. Accessed November 1, 2016.www.quran.com.

Ragheb, Seham, and Eleanor W. Smith. "Beliefs and customs regarding breast feeding among Egyptian women in Alexandria." *International Journal of Nursing Studies* 16 (1979): 73–83.

Ramzi Ismail, Saad. "The relationship between placental location and fetal gender (Ramzi's method)." Accessed November 15, 2016. http://www.obgyn.net/articles/relationship-between-placental-location-and-fetal-gender-ramzi%E2%80%99s-method.

Reiss, Rosemary E., and Avner D. Ash. "The eighth-month fetus: classical sources for a modern superstition." *Obstetrics & Gynecology* 71 (1988): 270–73.

Rempelakos, L., Costas Tsiamis, and E. Poulakou-Rebelakou. "Penile representations in ancient Greek art." *Archivos Espanoles de Urologia* 66 (2013): 911–16.

Richardson, A. Cullen, J. B. Lyon, E. E. Graham, and N. L. Williams. "Decreasing postpartum sexual abstinence time." *American Journal of Obstetrics & Gynecology* 126 (1976): 416–17.

Riddle, John M. "Artemisia, the 'mother herb.'" In *Goddesses, Elixirs, and Witches: Plants and Sexuality throughout Human History*, edited by John M. Riddle, 79–112. New York: Palgrave Macmillan, 2010.

———. *Contraception and Abortion From the Ancient World to the Renaissance*. Cambridge, MA: Harvard University Press, 1994.

Roberts, Christine L., Charles S. Algert, and Emily Olive. "Impact of first-stage ambulation on mode of delivery among women with epidural analgesia." *Australian and New Zealand Journal of Obstetrics & Gynaecology* 44 (2004): 489–94.

Roberts, Kathryn L, Maureen Reiter, and Diane Schuster. "A comparison of chilled and room temperature cabbage leaves in treating breast engorgement." *Journal of Human Lactation* 11 (1995): 191–94.

———. "Effects of cabbage leaf extract on breast engorgement." *Journal of Human Lactation* 14 (1998): 231–36.

Robertson, Sarah A., Leigh R. Guerin, Lachlan M. Moldenhauer, and John D. Hayball. "Activating T regulatory cells for tolerance in early pregnancy—the contribution of seminal fluid." *Journal of Reproductive Immunology* 83 (2009): 109–16.

Roemheld-Hamm, Beatrix. "Chasteberry." *American Family Physician* 72 (2005): 821–24.

Rosenzweig, Sanford. "Psychological stress in cleft palate etiology." *Journal of Dental Research* 6 Suppl (1966): 1585–93.

Roudsari, Robab Latifnejad, Helen T. Allan, and Pam A. Smith. "Looking at infertility through the lens of religion and spirituality: a review of the literature." *Human Fertility* 10 (2007): 141–49.

Rucker, M. Pierce. "An eighteenth century method of pain relief in obstetrics." *Journal of the History of Medicine* (1950): 101–5.

Ruegsegger Veit, Christina, and Raphael Jewelewicz. "Gender preselection: facts and myths." *Fertility and Sterility* 49 (1988): 937–40.

Sadler, Michael T. *The Law of Population*. London: John Murray, 1830.

Schaffir, Jonathan. "Birth rate and its correlation with the lunar cycle and specific atmospheric conditions." Letter to the editor. *American Journal of Obstetrics & Gynecology* 195 (2006): 878.

———. "Do patients associate adverse pregnancy outcomes with folkloric beliefs?" *Archives of Women's Mental Health* 10 (2007): 301–4.

———. "Sexual intercourse at term and onset of labor." *Obstetrics & Gynecology* 107 (2006): 1310–14.

———. "Survey of folk beliefs about induction of labor." *Birth* 29 (2002): 47–51.

————. "What are little boys made of? The never-ending search for sex selection techniques." *Perspectives in Biology and Medicine* 34 (1991): 516–25.

Schaffir, Jonathan, and Cheryl Czapla. "Survey of lactation instructors on folk traditions in breastfeeding." *Breastfeeding Medicine* 7 (2012): 230–33.

Schaffir, Jonathan, Alana McGee, and Elizabeth Kennard. "Use of nonmedical treatment by infertility patients." *Journal of Reproductive Medicine* 54 (2009): 415–20.

Schiff, Melissa A., Susan D. Reed, and Janet R. Daling, "The sex ratio of pregnancies complicated by hospitalisation for hyperemesis gravidarum," *British Journal of Obstetrics & Gynaecology* 111 (2004): 27–30.

Schlussel, Michaell Maia, Elton Bicalho deSouza, Michael Eduardo Reichenheim, and Gilberto Kac. "Physical activity during pregnancy and maternal-child health outcomes: a systematic literature review." *Cad Saude Publica* 24 Suppl 4 (2008): S531–44.

Selander, Jodi, Allison Cantor, Sharon M. Young, and Daniel C. Benyshek. "Human maternal placentophagy: a survey of self-reported motivations and experiences associated with placental consumption." *Ecology of Food and Nutrition* 52 (2013): 93–115.

Sha, Janet L. *Mothers of Thyme: Customs and Rituals of Infertility and Miscarriage.* Minneapolis: Lida Rose Press, 1990.

Shettles, Landrum B., and David M. Rorvik. *How to Choose the Sex of Your Baby.* New York: Doubleday, 1989.

Siega-Riz, Anna Maria, Tracy S. Herrmann, David A. Savitz, and John M. Thorp. "Frequency of eating during pregnancy and its effect on preterm delivery." *American Journal of Epidemiology* 153 (2001): 647–52.

Simcock, Barbara W. "Sons and daughters—a sex preselection study." *Medical Journal of Australia* 142 (1985): 541–42.

Simpson, Michele, Myra Parsons, Jennifer Greenwood, and Kenneth Wade. "Raspberry leaf in pregnancy: its safety and efficacy in labor." *Journal of Midwifery & Women's Health* 46 (2001): 51–59.

Smith, Caroline A., Carmel T. Collins, Allan M. Cyna, and Caroline A. Crowther. "Complemetary and alternative therapies for pain management in labour." *Cochrane Database of Systematic Reviews* 2006, Issue 4, Art No.: CD003521.

Smith, Caroline A., Kate M. Levett, Carmel T. Collins, and Caroline A. Crowther. "Relaxation techniques for pain management in labour." *Cochrane Database of Systematic Reviews* 2011, Issue 12, Art No.: CD009514.

Smith, J. Lewis. *A Treatise on the Diseases of Infancy and Childhood.* Philadelphia: Henry Lea, 1872.

Snapper, I. "Midwifery, past and present." *Bulletin of the New York Academy of Medicine* 39 (1963): 503–32.

Snow, Loudell F., Shirley M. Johnson, and Harry E. Mayhew. "The behavioral implications of some old wives' tales." *Obstetrics & Gynecology* 51 (1978): 727–32.

Sontag, L. W., and T. W. Richards. "Studies in fetal behavior: I. Fetal heart rate as a behavioral indicator." *Monographs of the Society for Research in Child Development* 3 (1938): 1–69.

Spacefem.com. "Due date statistics: a study on the length of pregnancy." Accessed November 8, 2016. http://spacefem.com/pregnant/charts/duedate6.php.

Speert, Harold. *Obstetrics and Gynecology: A History and Iconography.* San Francisco: Norman Publishing, 1994.

Spyropoulos, Evangelos, Dimitrios Borousas, Stamatios Mavrikos, Athanasios Dellis, Michael Bourounis, and Sotirios Athanasiadis. "Size of external genital organs and somatometric parameters among physically normal men younger than 40 years old." *Urology* 60 (2002): 485–89.

Stolkowski, Joseph, and Jacques Lorrain. "Preconceptional selection of fetal sex." *International Journal of Gynaecology and Obstetrics* 18 (1980): 440–43.

Tamimi, Rulla M., Pagona Lagiou, Lorelei A. Mucci, Chung-Cheng Hsieh, Hans-Olov Adami, and Dimitrios Trichopoulos. "Average energy intake among pregnant women carrying a boy compared with a girl." *BMJ: British Medical Journal* 326 (2003): 1245–46.

Tan, Peng Chiong, Choon Ming Yow, and Siti Zawiah Omar. "Effect of coital activity on onset of labor in women scheduled for labor induction: a randomized controlled trial." *Obstetrics & Gynecology* 110 (2007): 820–26.

Temkin, Owsei. *Soranus' Gynecology*. Baltimore: Johns Hopkins Press, 1956.

Terry, Samuel H. *Controlling Sex in Generation*. New York: Fowler & Wells, 1885.

Tezuka, Naohiro, Satoshi Sato, Michio Banzai, Hidekazu Saito, and Masahiko Hiroi. "Development and sexual difference in embryonic heart rates in pregnancies resulting from in vitro fertilization." *Gynecological and Obstetrical Investigation* 46 (1998): 217–19.

Tiemessen, Carolina H. J., Johannes L. H. Evers, and Robert S. G. M. Bots. "Tight-fitting underwear and sperm quality." *Lancet* 347 (1996): 1844–45.

Tiran, Denise. "Use of pineapple for induction of labour." *The Practising Midwife* 12 (2009): 33–34.

Todman, Donald. "Childbirth in ancient Rome: from traditional folklore to obstetrics." *Australian and New Zealand Journal of Obstetrics & Gynaecology* 47 (2007): 82–85.

Vatten, Lars J., and Rolv Skjaerven. "Offspring sex and pregnancy outcome by length of gestation." *Early Human Development* 76 (2004): 47–54.

Walker, Molly Kay, and Garris Keels Conner. "Fetal sex preference of second-trimester gravidas." *Journal of Nurse-Midwifery* 38 (1993): 110–13.

Wall, L. Lewis. "The strange case of Mary Toft (who was delivered of sixteen rabbits and a tabby cat in 1726)." *Medical Heritage* 3 (1985): 199–212.

Walter, Marie. "The folklore of breastfeeding." *Bulletin of the New York Academy of Medicine* 51 (1975): 870–76.

Warkany, Josef, and Harold Kalter. "Maternal impressions and congenital malformations." *Plastic and Reconstructive Surgery* 30 (1962): 628–37.

Westphal, Lynn M., Mary L. Polan, and Aileen S. Trant. "Double-blind, placebo-controlled study of Fertilityblend: a nutritional supplement for improving fertility in women." *Clinical Experiments in Obstetrics and Gynecology* 33 (2006): 205–8.

Whelan, Elizabeth M. *Boy or Girl? The Sex Selection Technique That Makes All Others Obsolete*. Indianapolis: Bobbs-Merrill, 1978.

Wilcox, Allen J., Clarice R. Weinberg, and Donna D. Baird. "Timing of sexual intercourse in relation to ovulation." *New England Journal of Medicine* 333 (1995): 1517–21.

Williams, J. Whitridge. *Obstetrics: a Textbook for the Use of Students and Practitioners*. 6th ed. New York: Appleton & Co., 1930.

Wilson, Philip K. "'Out of sight, out of mind?': the Daniel Turner–James Blondel dispute over the power of the maternal imagination." *Annals of Science* 49 (1992): 63–85.

Woywodt, Alexander, and Akos Kiss. "Geophagia: the history of earth-eating." *Journal of the Royal Society of Medicine* 95 (2002): 143–46.

Young, Sera L. "Pica in pregnancy: new ideas about an old condition." *Annual Review of Nutrition* 30 (2010): 403–22.

Zisk, Jody L., Linda H. Genen, Sharon Kirkby, David Webb, Jay Greenspan, and Kevin Dysart. "Do premature female infants really do better than their male counterparts?" *American Journal of Perinatology* 28 (2011): 241–46.

Zuppa, Antonio Alberto, Paola Sindico, Claudia Orchi, Chiara Carducci, Valentina Cardiello, Costantino Romagnoli, and Piero Catenazzi. "Safety and efficacy of galactogogues: substances that induce, maintain and increase breast milk production." *Journal of Pharmacy and Pharmaceutical Sciences* 13 (2010): 162–74.

WEBOGRAPHY

The following is a list of websites offering discussions and pregnancy recommendations. It is not meant to be exhaustive, since these websites seem to pop up and change at short intervals. It is also not meant to be an endorsement of any of the views or opinions provided in them. For readers interested in seeing the kinds of recommendations and folklore that are widely circulated on the Internet and that have inspired this book, the list is a jumping off point to explore the wide range of offerings found on the web.

www.aboutamom.com
www.babiesonline.com
www.babycenter.com
www.babycentre.co.uk
www.babygaga.com
www.bellybelly.com
www.cafemom.com
www.circleofmoms.com
www.fitpregnancy.com
www.fortunebaby.com
www.ingender.com
www.justmommies.com
www.kidspot.com.au/birth
www.mamaseeds.com
www.matrika-india.org
www.momforum.com

www.momtastic.com/pregnancy
www.motherandbaby.co.uk
www.mothercare.com
www.newkidscenter.com/pregnancy
www.parenting.com
www.parents.com
www.pregnancy.org
www.pregnancyweekly.com
www.pregnantchicken.com
www.romper.com
www.sheknows.com
www.storknet.com
www.thebump.com
www.thegenderexperts.com
www.theempoweredmomma.com
www.todaysparent.com/pregnancy
www.whattoexpect.com

INDEX

ABOUT THE AUTHOR

Jonathan Schaffir, MD, is a practicing obstetrician, with over twenty-five years of experience caring for pregnant women and delivering babies. He is also a medical educator and faculty member at the Ohio State University College of Medicine. He is a past president of the North American Society for Psychosocial Obstetrics and Gynecology, an interdisciplinary society that brings together various professionals who have interests in sociocultural and psychological aspects of obstetrics and women's health. With extensive experience researching and writing in the field of obstetrical folklore, Schaffir's work has been cited in major magazines such as *Parents, American Baby, Self,* and *Child.* He has also appeared on local news programs to comment on recently published studies of obstetrics folklore.